Atlas of Nail Signs and Disorders with Clinical and Onychoscopic Correlation

This atlas allows dermatologists and resident and qualified professionals in other disciplines to reach a quick diagnosis, with a wealth of clinical and dermatoscopic images for convenience.

Key features:

- Provides a quick and straightforward guide to diagnosis for medical professionals.
- Allows residents and professionals in other disciplines easy access to the essential points.
- Presents the expertise of some of the most eminent international nail specialists.

Nilton Di Chiacchio is Head of the Dermatologic Clinic, Hospital do Servidor Público Municipal de São Paulo, São Paulo, Brazil.

Nilton Gioia Di Chiacchio is a dermatologist at Faculdade de Medicina do ABC, São André, and Hospital do Servidor Público Municipal de São Paulo, São Paulo, Brazil.

Robertha Carvalho de Nakamura is a dermatologist at Instituto di Dermatologia, Santa Casa da Misericordia, Rio de Janeiro, Brazil.

Michela Starace is a dermatologist at IRCCS Azienda Ospedaliero-Universitaria di Bologna and Assistant Professor at Alma Mater Studiorum, University of Bologna, Italy.

Matilde Iorizzo is a dermatologist in private practice (Bellinzona and Lugano, Switzerland); she is also the Vice President of the European Nail Society and the Secretary of the International Nail Society.

Robert Baran is Head of the Nail Disease Center in Cannes, France; *Baran and Dawber's Diseases of the Nails and their Management* is now in its fifth edition.

Atlas of Nail Signs and Disorders with Clinical and Onychoscopic Correlation

Nilton Di Chiacchio, MD
Head of the Dermatologic Clinic
Hospital do Servidor Público Municipal de São Paulo
São Paulo, Brazil

Nilton Gioia Di Chiacchio, MD, PhD
Dermatologist at Faculdade de Medicina do ABC São André
Hospital do Servidor Público Municipal de São Paulo
São Paulo, Brazil

Robertha Carvalho de Nakamura, MS, MD
Dermatologist at Institute of Dermatology
Santa Casa da Misericordia
Rio de Janeiro, Brazil

Michela Starace, MD, PhD
Dermatologist at IRCCS Azienda Ospedaliero-Universitaria di Bologna
Assistant Professor at Alma Mater Studiorum
University of Bologna
Bologna, Italy

Matilde Iorizzo, MD, PhD
Dermatologist in private practice
Bellinzona and Lugano, Switzerland

Robert Baran, MD
Head of the Nail Disease Center
Cannes, France

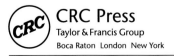

CRC Press
Taylor & Francis Group
Boca Raton London New York

CRC Press is an imprint of the
Taylor & Francis Group, an **informa** business

Designed cover image: Author

First edition published 2024
by CRC Press
2385 NW Executive Center Drive, Suite 320, Boca Raton FL 33431

and by CRC Press
4 Park Square, Milton Park, Abingdon, Oxon, OX14 4RN

CRC Press is an imprint of Taylor & Francis Group, LLC

ISBN: 978-1-032-25790-7 (hbk)
ISBN: 978-1-032-25786-0 (pbk)
ISBN: 978-1-003-28502-1 (ebk)

DOI: 10.1201/b22852

Typeset in Minion Pro
by KnowledgeWorks Global Ltd.

Contents

I

Nail Signs

CHAPTER 1

Anatomy

ANATOMICAL STRUCTURES OF THE NAIL UNIT

Knowledge of the nail unit structures is essential to perform a proper physical and dermoscopic examination.

The nail unit occupies the dorsal aspect of the last phalanx of the digits and comprises the nail matrix, nail bed, nail plate, proximal fold, lateral folds, and distal sulcus. The nail plate is produced by the nail matrix and bed: They are all intimately connected by cuticular or corneal components (**Figures 1.1** and **1.2**). In the proximal region, the proximal fold produces the cuticle at its free end, which secures and adheres the proximal nail fold to the dorsal nail plate. The cuticle acts as a physical barrier protecting the matrix from infiltration of infectious organisms, allergens, or irritants. The lateral folds also frame and protect the nail plate. The onychodermal band, located at the distal subungual region, is the last point of adherence of the nail plate to the bed. Finally, the hyponychium is a specialized keratinized structure that forms the distal nail groove and seals the subungual space. The distal grove is the cutaneous ridge demarcating the border between subungual structures

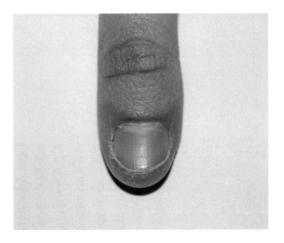

FIGURE 1.1   Clinical picture of normal fingernail.

DOI: 10.1201/b22852-2

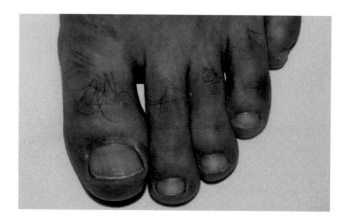

FIGURE 1.2   Clinical picture of normal toenail.

and the finger pulp. This region is favorable for the formation of a known reservoir for various microorganisms, often responsible for secondary changes in the nail plate. The epithelium of the hyponychium is highly vascularized and highly vulnerable to bleeding and pain with a minimal trauma.

Definition of anatomical structures of the nail unit:

- *Nail plate*: Keratinized, hard, semi-transparent structure that grows continuously throughout life.

- *Lateral nail folds*: Lateral cutaneous folds that frame the lateral borders of the nail plate.

- *Proximal nail folds*: Proximal cutaneous fold covered with epithelium in its ventral and dorsal surfaces and forming the cuticle in its free end. The ventral surface of the proximal fold forms the eponychium region. Below this structure is located the proximal matrix.

- *Cuticle*: Epidermal layer, produced by the ventral region of the proximal fold and firmly adherent to the dorsal surface of the nail plate (**Figures 1.3** and **1.4**).

- *Nail matrix*: It can be divided into three parts. The dorsal or proximal matrix that is located below the proximal fold and morphologically is oblique and responsible for the formation of the dorsal nail plate surface. The intermediate, germinal, or distal matrix

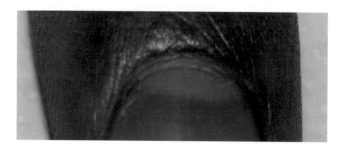

FIGURE 1.3   Clinical picture of the cuticle.

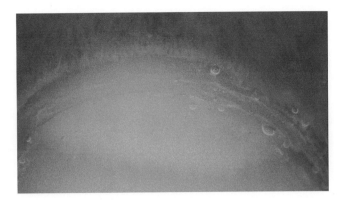

FIGURE 1.4   Onychoscopy picture of the cuticle (40x).

begins when the dorsal matrix folds on itself. It produces most of the nail plate (80% approximately) and, in particular, the intermediate and hardest region of the nail plate. The ventral matrix, or nail bed, begins where the intermediate matrix ends and extends to the onychodermal band. In its proximal region, it has two lateral horns or ridges.

- *Lunula (half-moon)*: The convex edge of the intermediate or distal matrix, seen through the nail plate. It is whitish, contrasting with the color of the adjacent nail bed; it is most commonly visible on the thumbs and big toenails; and its appearance decreases in the subsequent fingers/toes (**Figure 1.5**).

- *Nail bed, ventral matrix, or sterile matrix*: Vascular bed on which the nail plate rests. It extends from the lunula to the onychodermal band. It has a striated shape, has the function of adhesion, and helps the continuous movement of the nail plate. Nail bed can be observed with the dermoscope through the nail plate, taking care not to push the lens too hard in order to not cause bleaching of the nail bed vasculature. Magnifications required range from 10x to 40x.

- *Onychodermal band*: It is a transverse band located in the distal region of the nail bed. Its color is different from the nail bed (pink, white, or brown, depending on

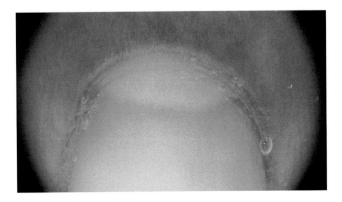

FIGURE 1.5   Onychoscopy picture of the lunula (20x).

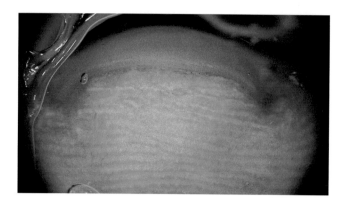

FIGURE 1.6   Onychoscopy picture of the distal margin (20x).

the skin color of each patient). It is the region of greatest adherence of the nail plate before physiological onycholysis and represents the first barrier against penetration by microorganisms, irritants, or foreign bodies.

- *Hyponychium*: It corresponds to the epidermis of the subungual region of the distal physiological onycholysis (nail plate free edge) and it is limited by the distal sulcus and produces its distal horny layer (**Figures 1.6** and **1.7**).

- *Distal sulcus*: It is present in the distal region of the hyponychium and limits the end of the nail bed with the local skin structure.

The fingers are supplied by four arteries derived from the superficial and deep palmar arches: two on each side, the dorsal and palmar or plantar arteries. When they reach the nail unit, in the distal region of the finger, they form a superficial arcade immediately after the distal phalanx and provide blood flow for the nail fold and matrix. The subungual region is supplied by the proximal and distal subungual arcades, arising from anastomoses of the palmar arcade and the superficial arcade. Venous drainage from the finger through deep and superficial systems is similar. The nail bed is richly supplied with glomus bodies: neurovascular bodies that act as arteriovenous anastomoses. They are

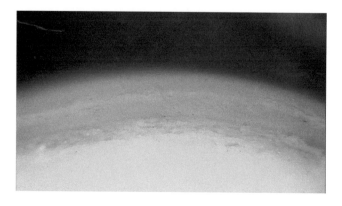

FIGURE 1.7   Onychoscopy picture of the distal margin (40x).

FIGURE 1.8 Onychoscopy picture of the normal capillary network of periungual tissue (capillaroscopy) (40x).

regulators of peripheral capillary circulation in cold conditions. The capillary network of the nail fold is easily seen with the dermoscope, better at high magnification (50–70x) and with use of an interface solution (ultrasound gel). The capillary loops are horizontal and visible along their entire length. The loops are in layers of uniform size, with peaks equidistant from the base of the cuticle. Capillary density is considered normal if the number of capillaries exceeds 9 per linear mm (average range: 9–12 capillaries per mm) (**Figure 1.8**).

The nail unit is innervated by the median, ulnar, and radial nerves in its dorsal and palmar or plantar portions. The median nerve supplies the nail unit of the first, second, third, and lateral of the fourth fingers. The ulnar nerve innervates the lateral portion of the fourth and fifth fingers, and the radial nerve innervates the lateral portion of the first finger.

The extensor tendon is located on the dorsum of the distal phalanx, intimately connected to the nail unit. The lateral tendon is positioned on the subungual sides attached to the distal region of the distal phalanx.

SUGGESTED READINGS

Canavan TN, Graham LV, Elewski BE. Subungual space: The next frontier. *Skin Appendage Disord.* 2018;5:50–51.

De Berker D. Nail anatomy. *Clin Dermatol.* 2013;31(5):509–515.

De Berker D, Ruben BS, Baran R. Science of the nail apparatus. In Baran R, De Berker D, Holzberg M, Piraccini BM, Richert B, Thomas L, eds. *Baran & Dawber's Diseases of the Nails and Their Management*, 5th edn. Chichester, West Sussex: John Wiley & Sons Ltd; 2019: 1–26.

Garson JC, Baltenneck F, Leroy F, et al. Histological structure of human nail as studied by synchrotron X-ray microdiffraction. *Cell Mol Biol.* 2000;46:1025–1034.

González-Serva. Normal nail anatomy. In Rubin AI, Jellinek NJ, Daniel CR III, Scher RK, eds. *Scher and Daniel's Nails: Diagnosis, Surgery, Therapy*, 4th edn. Oxford, UK: Springer; 2018: 41–56.

Haneke E. Anatomy of the nail unit and the nail biopsy. *Semin Cutan Med Surg.* 2015;34(2):95–100.

Haneke E., ed. Development, structure, and function of the nail. *Histopathology of the Nail: Onychopathology*. Boca Raton, FL: CRC Press; 2017: 1–18.

Nail Dermoscopy. Starace M (2018) In: Sher and Daniel's Nails. Diagnosis, Surgery, Therapy. Rubin A, Jellinek N, Ralph Daniel III C, Scher RK. ISBN: 978-3-319-65647-2, doi: 10.1007/978-3-319-65649-6

Zaias N. Anatomy and physiology. *The Nail in Health and Disease*. Jamaica: SP Medical and Scientific Books; 1980: 1–18. DOI: 10.1007/978-94-011-7846-4_1

CHAPTER 2

Nail Matrix Signs

ONYCHORREXIS AND ONYCHOSCHIZIA

Onychorrexis describes a split at the free edge of the nail plate that extends proximally. The nail plate is usually thin and presents furrows running parallel to the split in the superficial layers. Multiple splits can be observed (**Figure 2.1**).

Onychoschizia is a lamellar exfoliation into fine horizontal layers of the distal portion of the nail plate (**Figure 2.2**).

They are both typical signs of nail fragility affecting the distal portion of the nail plate. Patients often complain of cosmetic and functional problems, but rarely pain. Affected plates are weak and with a reduced elasticity—this is why they split. Fragility is associated

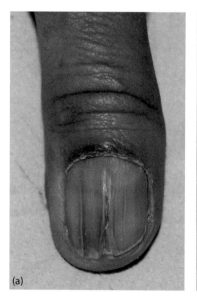 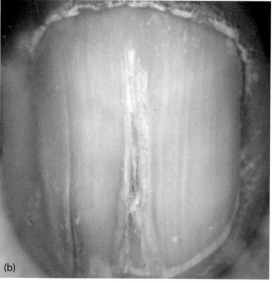

(a) (b)

FIGURE 2.1   (a) Clinical picture: onychorrhexis or parallel longitudinal grooves at different degrees of depth. (b) Onychoscopy: shallow and deep longitudinal grooves, observe the separation of the dorsal nail plate, with the ventral nail plate remaining visible.

   DOI: 10.1201/b22852-3

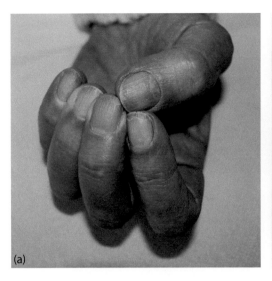
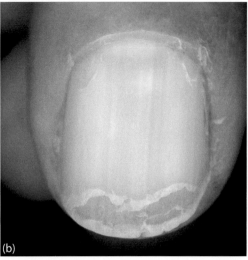

FIGURE 2.2   (a) Clinical and (b) onychoscopy pictures of onychoschizia.

with a defect in the intercellular cement that holds together nail plate keratinocytes and with a disorganized protein and lipid structure (dishomogeneous orientation of keratin filaments and reduced lipid content). This may be due to age or may be secondary to dermatological (lichen planus and trachyonychia for example) or systemic diseases (amyloidosis for example), nutritional deficiencies, traumas, and drug intake. Possible etiology is very important, especially in the elderly population, where many comorbidities can be present as well as multiple drug intake.

BEAU'S LINE AND ONYCHOMADESIS

Beau's line describes a transverse depression on the nail plate surface due to a mild interference, a transitory arrest, with nail plate formation (**Figure 2.3**).

Onychomadesis describes the detachment of the nail plate from the proximal nail fold with the formation of a transverse whole-thickness sulcus. It is due to a severe

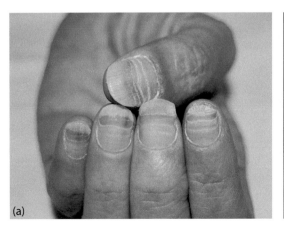
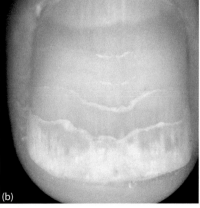

FIGURE 2.3   (a) Clinical and (b) onychoscopy pictures of Beau's line.

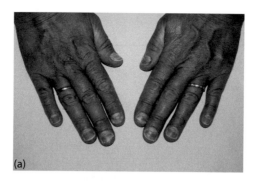

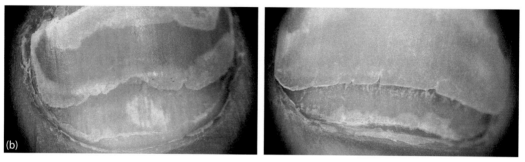

FIGURE 2.4   (a) Clinical and (b) onychoscopy pictures of onychomadesis.

insult producing complete arrest of nail plate production, and it is considered a progression of a severe Beau's line. Such a full-thickness sulcus usually leads to nail plate loss.

Both are deeper in the central portion of the nail plate and move distally with nail growth. They become visible on the nail plate surface usually some weeks after the insult.

Insults repeated over time produce multiple grooves on the same plate. The distance of each groove from the nail fold is related to the time since the onset of the insult. When several digits are involved, this may indicate a systemic condition (**Figure 2.4**).

PITTING

Pits are punctate depression of the nail plate surface due to defective keratinization of the proximal nail matrix with the production of clusters of parakeratotic cells (nucleated and incompletely keratinized) in the dorsal nail plate. These clusters are easily detached at minimal trauma, leaving superficial holes (pits) that migrate distally with nail growth.

Pitting is commonly seen in nail psoriasis and in alopecia areata. In nail psoriasis pits are typically large, deep, irregular in size, and randomly distributed (**Figure 2.5**). In alopecia areata of the nails, pits are more regular in size and geometrically distributed (**Figure 2.6**).

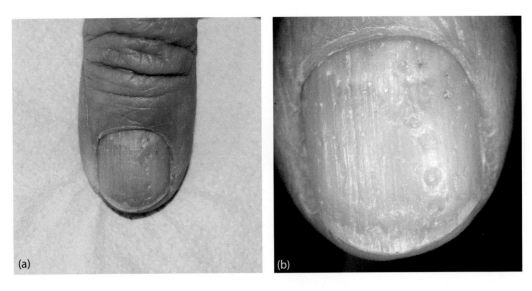

FIGURE 2.5   (a) Clinical and (b) onychoscopy pictures of irregular pitting.

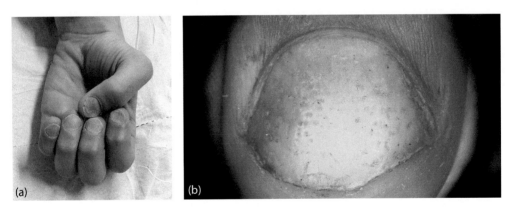

FIGURE 2.6   (a) Clinical and (b) onychoscopy pictures of regular pitting.

TRACHYONYCHIA

Trachyonychia, formerly known as 20-nail dystrophy, presents as brittle, rough (*sandpapered*), and opaque nail plates. This is due to severe and persistent inflammation to the proximal nail matrix. The inflammation could also be milder and intermittent, and the result is a shiny variant. The two variants may coexist in the same patient. Trachyonychia usually affects all 20 nails, but it can affect also just one plate (**Figures 2.7** and **2.8**).

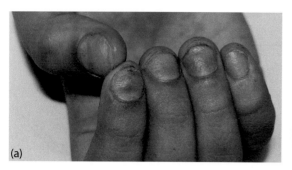 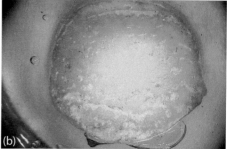

FIGURE 2.7 (a) Clinical and (b) onychoscopy pictures of opaque trachyonychia.

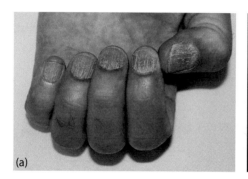 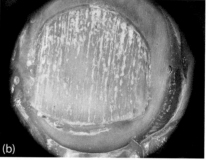

FIGURE 2.8 (a) Clinical and (b) onychoscopy pictures of shiny trachyonychia.

It is most commonly seen in children and usually improves over time even without treatment. Trachyonychia is not a distinctive disorder, but it is the clinical result of disorders that involve the nail matrix. Diagnosis of the causative disease always requires a biopsy. It is mainly associated with alopecia areata, eczema, psoriasis, and lichen planus, but it can also be idiopathic.

PACHYONYCHIA

Pachyonychia means a thickened, opaque, and yellowish nail plate with an increased transverse curvature (**Figure 2.9**). The growth rate is reduced, and nail trimming is extremely difficult. Trauma and impaired blood supply are probable predisposing factors for this onychodystrophy in the elderly. The repeated constraints between shoes and toes are also possible culprits. Genetic mutations are instead responsible for the congenital forms (pachyonychia congenita).

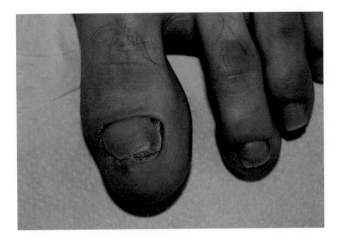

FIGURE 2.9   Clinical picture of pachyonychia.

ONYCHOGRYPHOSIS

The nail plate is typically thickened, elevated, with transverse ridges on its surface, as one side of the plate grows faster than the other (**Figure 2.10**). The side that grows faster determines the direction of the plate. The big toenail of elderly people has frequently this shape. Other toenails may also be affected. Predisposing factors include trauma, ill-fitting shoes, impaired blood supply, and poor foot care.

CHROMONYCHIA

Chromonychia means an abnormality of color affecting the nail plate. The pigment may be of endogenous or of exogenous origin. We will discuss here cases of pigment originating from the nail matrix.

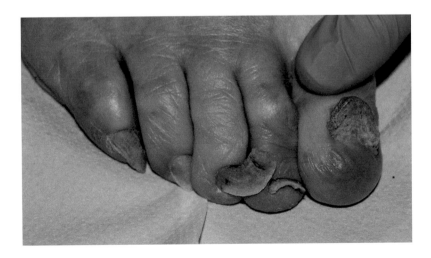

FIGURE 2.10   Clinical picture of onychogryphosis.

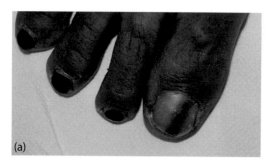
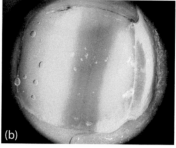

FIGURE 2.11   (a) Clinical and (b) onychoscopy pictures of melanonychia due to nevus.

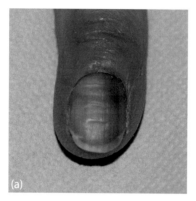
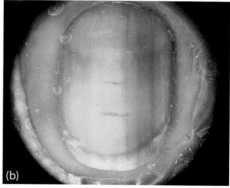

FIGURE 2.12   (a) Clinical and (b) onychoscopy pictures of melanonychia due to traumatic melanocytic activation.

Melanonychia describes the presence of melanin within the nail plate (**Figures 2.11–2.14**). When the production of melanin originates from nail matrix cells, melanonychia present as a longitudinal band extending from the nail matrix to the nail plate free edge. The nail plate may show different shades of brown, black, and grey. The entire plate can be involved.

Production of melanin can be due to melanocyte activation (ethnicity, drug intake, inflammatory/infective disorder), a benign (lentigo, nevus), or malignant melanocyte

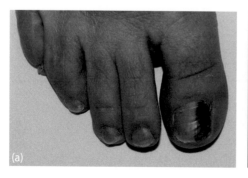
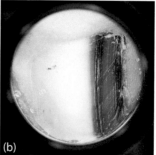

FIGURE 2.13   (a) Clinical and (b) onychoscopy pictures of melanonychia due to melanoma *in situ*.

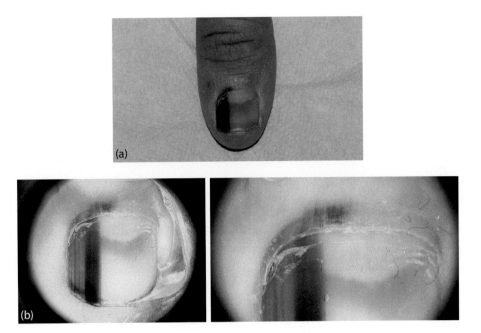

FIGURE 2.14   (a) Clinical and (b) onychoscopy pictures of melanonychia due to melanoma *in situ*.

hyperplasia (melanoma). Pigmented tumors originating from the matrix can also be responsible for melanonychia.

Melanonychia can involve one digit or several digits, both in fingernails and toenails, and it can occur at any age. The number of digits involved is an important diagnostic clue. If more than one digit is involved, the first thought should be an activation.

Dermoscopy of melanocytic nail pigmentation is however sometimes difficult to interpret, as there are still not uniform criteria that allow us to differentiate melanonychia due to benign melanocytic proliferation, as nail matrix lentigo or nevus, from melanonychia due to malignant melanocytic proliferation. The real problem is that with the dermoscope we cannot observe the origin of the pigment but only its deposition within the plate.

Observing the nail plate free edge, with the aid of a dermoscope, we can instead establish the origin of the pigment. If the pigment is located in the upper portion of the free edge, the source is likely to be the proximal portion of the matrix; if the pigment is found in the lower portion, it favors a more distal matrix location.

A more detailed description of the melanic bands will be provided in the specific chapter in the second part of this book.

Histologically, melanonychia can then be due to melanocytic activation or proliferation (lentigo, nevi, melanoma). Melanonychia caused by melanocyte activation often involves several nails and is a more common occurrence in patients with darker skin phototypes. Activation can also be due to drugs, inflammation, and endocrine disorders.

Infections and tumors may also be responsible of activation.

Cyanonychia means blue nails and when the origin is the matrix, the culprits are usually nutritional deficiencies or adverse reaction to drugs.

Nail changes in vitamin B12 deficiency are common. They present a bluish discoloration, bluish-black pigmentation with dark longitudinal streaks, and darkened longitudinal and reticulate streaks. They are more frequent in dark-skinned patients. The mechanism of hyperpigmentation is thought to be a decrease in glutathione levels, resulting in disinhibition of tyrosinase, a melanogenesis enzyme that leads to increased melanin synthesis. Nail discoloration due to drugs has some postulated mechanisms including melanocyte stimulation, deposition of drug metabolite, and drug-induced immune dysregulation leading to melanin pigment incontinence. Some examples are chloroquine and silver (argyria) inducing dark blue nail. Zidovudine therapy, and more rarely Imatinib, also produces dark blue nails in adults and children. This blue discoloration of the nails seems to be reversible and comparatively dose-dependent.

Erythronychia indicates one or multiple longitudinal red streaks along the nail plate (**Figures 2.15** and **2.16**). In correspondence with the streaks, the nail plate is thinner and the bed vessels are more visible—this is why the streaks appear red in color. Distal nail

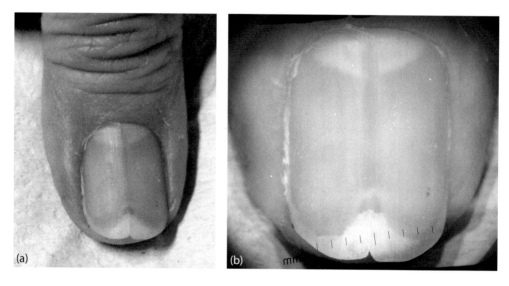

FIGURE 2.15   (a) Clinical and (b) onychoscopy pictures of one single band of erythronychia.

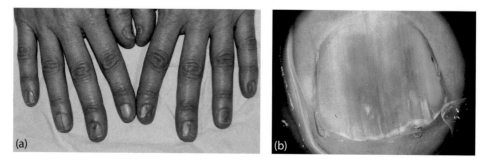

FIGURE 2.16   (a) Clinical and (b) onychoscopy pictures of multiple bands of erythronychia.

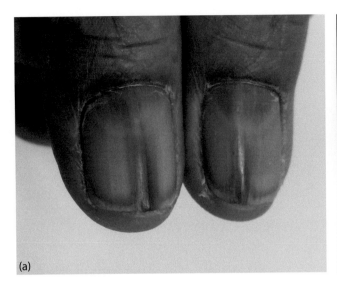
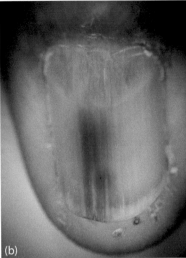

FIGURE 2.17 (a) Clinical and (b) onychoscopy pictures of diffuse erythronychia in the region of the lunula.

plate splitting may be associated. Multiple streaks usually indicate an inflammatory nail disorder (lichen planus and Darier disease most commonly), and a single streak is usually due to a benign tumor (onychopapilloma), but malignant tumors (Bowen, squamous cell carcinoma) have been reported as well. Where no primary disease can be identified to explain erythronychia affecting multiple nails, the descriptive term 'idiopathic polydactylous erythronychia' has been proposed.

The lunular area may also show diffuse or patchy erythematous color (**Figure 2.17**). Red lunulae may be a consequence of inflammatory disorders affecting the vessels of the distal nail matrix. Erythema of all, or part of the lunula, may affect all digits, but it is usually most prominent in the thumb.

Leukonychia means white nails. When the nail plate is entirely white or white in spots, longitudinal or transverse bands that do not fade with pressure, we are facing true leukonychia due to matrix abnormalities. The white color is due to the presence of parakeratotic cells within the nail plate that move distally with the plate growth.

Leukonychia can be temporary or permanent, monodactylous or polydactylous.

Obviously, monodactylous leukonychia most likely is caused by local factors involving that digit, while polydactylous indicates a systemic factor. Leukonychia is usually not an alarming sign, but it can sometimes unmask severe systemic disorders or congenital conditions. Congenital partial or total leukonychia is the most difficult to diagnose; it may exist as an isolated feature, or in association with other cutaneous or systemic pathologies as well as syndromes associated with sensorineural deafness (the GJB2 gene located on chromosome 13 encodes for connexin 26 which is responsible about half of cases of inherited sensorineural deafness).

Xanthonychia means yellow nail. The nail plate color becomes yellow in the yellow nail syndrome (see chapter) where fingernails and toenails are excessively curved from side to side and cuticles are usually absent as well as the lunula. The growth rate is reduced. It is an

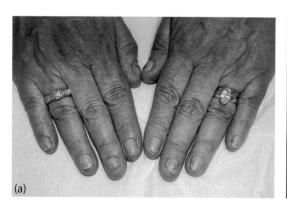
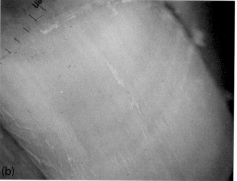

FIGURE 2.18   (a) Clinical and (b) onychoscopy pictures of yellow nail sydrome.

acquired condition of unknown etiology characterized by a triad of thickened and yellow-ish nails, primary lymphedema, and respiratory manifestations.

Yellow nails have also been described in lichen planus, especially in the toenails. Typical lichen planus of the fingernails usually helps in the differential diagnosis (**Figure 2.18**).

ANONYCHIA AND MICRONYCHIA

It means the absence of the nail plate or nail plate reduced size (**Figure 2.19**). It may be congenital or acquired. The most common congenital causes of anonychia/micronychia are alcohol abuse or drugs taken by the mother during the first months of pregnancy (anticonvulsants, anticoagulants, morphine above all), Iso–Kikuchy syndrome, nail-patella syndrome, DOOR syndrome, and some ectodermal dysplasias. In some instances, underlying bone may be involved so performing an X-ray is highly recommended.

Acquired micronychia results from total or partial destruction of the nail matrix due to inflammatory disorders or trauma. Among inflammatory disorders, the most common

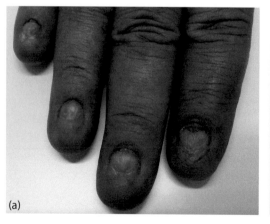
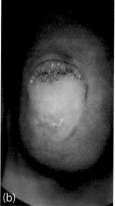
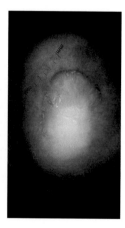

FIGURE 2.19   (a) Clinical and (b) onychoscopy pictures of anonychia/micronychia.

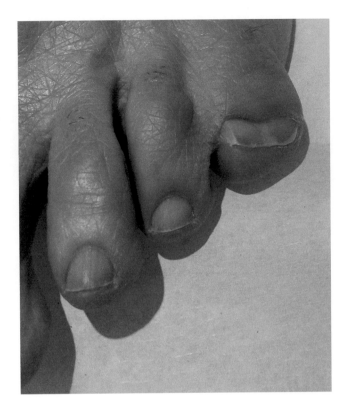

FIGURE 2.20   Clinical picture of macronychia.

cause is nail lichen planus in its severe form. Depending on the severity of the disease, micronychia can progress to anonychia (no nail plate). Apparent micronychia may be due to overlapping of the nail surface by thick lateral nail folds, as in Turner syndrome and chronic recalcitrant paronychia.

MACRONYCHIA

Nails are larger than normal and affect one or more fingers with enlargement of the nail bed and/or matrix areas (**Figure 2.20**). They may occur in association with megadactyly, epiloia, Proteus syndrome, Maffucci syndrome, and Klippel–Trénaunay–Weber syndrome. It is seen in duplication of the distal phalanx, accompanied by a broad finger with a bivalved nail, fissured, or confluent nail. Macronychia can be seen in pseudomegadactyly and appears as a hypertrophy of the nail plate and bed due to a chronic granulomatous paronychia.

DOLICHONYCHIA

Dolichonychia is a descriptive term for nails that are long in length and short in width.

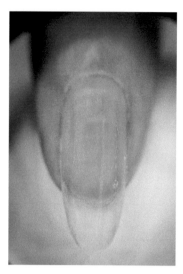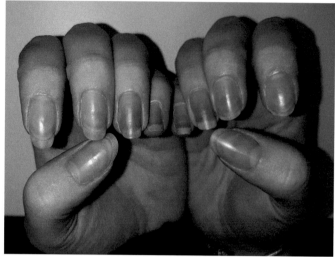

FIGURE 2.21   Clinical pictures of dolichonychia.

This clinical feature may be observed in patients with Ehlers–Danlos syndrome, hypohidrotic ectodermal dysplasia, Marfan syndrome, hypopituitarism, and in persons with eunuchoidism (**Figure 2.21**).

BRACHYONYCHIA

In brachyonychia, short nails or "racket nails," the width of the nail plate (and the nail bed) is greater than the length. It may occur in isolation or associated with a shortening of the terminal phalanx (**Figure 2.22**). Brachyonychia can be inherited as an autosomal dominant trait and is typically limited to the thumb but may involve multiple nails. It can be a defect in the closure of the epiphysis of the terminal phalanx of the thumb. This condition

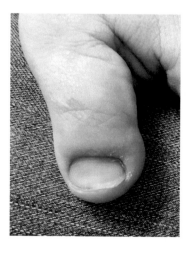

FIGURE 2.22   Clinical picture of brachyonychia.

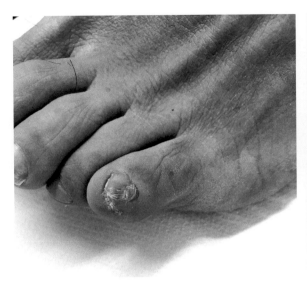
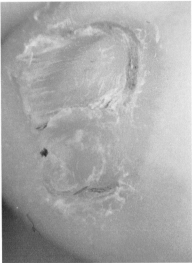

FIGURE 2.23   Onychoscopy picture of double nail of the fifth toe.

has been reported in association with brachydactyly, mental retardation, Spiegler tumors, cartilage–hair hypoplasia, acroosteolysis, Larsen syndrome, and acrodysostosis. Acquired racquet nails have been associated with hyperparathyroidism with resorption of the distal terminal phalanges and psoriatic arthropathy and nail biting.

DOUBLE NAIL OF THE FIFTH TOE

It is a rare onychodysplasia with variable genetic expression. It can be congenital, hereditary, or acquired. The nail plate is apparently divided into two parts by an intermediate groove. The medial plate is usually larger than the lateral one (**Figure 2.23**). Y-shaped radiological changes of the distal phalanx were occasionally detected. Some authors consider it a variation of the ectopic nail.

Among the associations described in the literature are the feeling of discomfort, a clubfoot with external rotation of the little toe, and a circumscribed callus lateral to the nail.

SUGGESTED READINGS

Apalla Z, Sotiriou E, Pikou O, et al. Onychomadesis after hand-foot-and-mouth disease outbreak in northern Greece: case series and brief review of the literature. *Int J Dermatol.* 2015;54(9):1039–44.

Chelidze K, Lipner SR. Nail changes in alopecia areata: an update and review. *Int J Dermatol.* 2018;57(7):776–83.

Chessa MA, Iorizzo M, Richert B, et al. Pathogenesis, clinical signs and treatment recommendations in brittle nails: a review. *Dermatol Ther (Heidelb).* 2020;10(1):15–27.

de Berker DAR. What is a Beau's line? *Int J Dermatol.* 1994;33(8):545–6.

Haneke E. Double nail of the little toe. *Skin Appendage Disord.* 2016;1(4):163–7.

Haneke E. Nail psoriasis: clinical features, pathogenesis, differential diagnoses, and management. *Psoriasis (Auckl).* 2017;7:51–63.

Hardin J, Haber RM. Onychomadesis: literature review. *Br J Dermatol.* 2015;172(2):592–6.

Inthasot S, André J, Richert B. Causes of longitudinal nail splitting: a retrospective 56-case series with clinical pathological correlation. *J Eur Acad Dermatol Venereol.* 2022;36(5):744–53.

Iorizzo M, Starace M, Pasch MC. Leukonychia: What can white nails tell us? *Am J Clin Dermatol.* 2022;23(2):177–93.

Jellinek NJ. Longitudinal erythronychia: suggestions for evaluation and management. *J Am Acad Dermatol.* 2011;64(1):167.e1–11.

Moffitt DL, de Berker DA. Yellow nail syndrome: the nail that grows half as fast grows twice as thick. *Clin Exp Dermatol.* 2000;25(1):21–3.

Starace M, Bruni F, Alessandrini A, Piraccini BM. Trachyonychia: a retrospective study of 122 patients in a period of 30 years. *J Eur Acad Dermatol Venereol.* 2020;34(4):880–4.

Tosti A, Piraccini BM, de Farias DC. Dealing with melanonychia. *Semin Cutan Med Surg.* 2009;28(1):49–54.

Nail Bed Signs

ONYCHOLYSIS

Onycholysis means separation of the nail plate from the underlying nail bed due to disruption of the onychocorneal band. It generally starts at the distal free margin of the nail plate and progresses proximally. Less often, it happens the other way around. Onycholysis is easily diagnosed clinically as a whitish appearance of the detached plate due to the light reflecting through it. Dermoscopy is extremely helpful to differentiate traumatic onycholysis from onycholysis due to other causes, mainly onychomycosis, and psoriasis. In traumatic onycholysis, the line of detachment is linear, regular and smooth, and surrounded by a normally pale pink-bed, without hyperkeratosis. In psoriasis the margin is slightly dented with orange-yellow border that corresponds to the clinical erythematous borders surrounding the distal edge of the detached nail plate. In onychomycoses, onycholysis has a ragged border due to the striped shapes of fungi invasion (**Figures 3.1–3.4**).

Onycholysis may be idiopathic, traumatic, or secondary to nail bed disorders. The majority of cases are due to physical trauma as improper nail care and mechanical abnormalities during gait (abnormal gait, poor fitting shoes). Traumatic working conditions, subungual masses, and dermatological diseases such as psoriasis, lichen planus, and

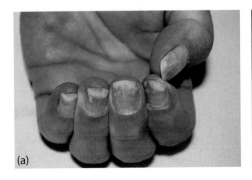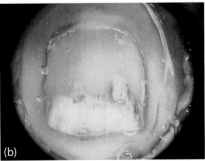

FIGURE 3.1   (a) Clinical and (b) onychoscopy of simple onycholysis.

DOI: 10.1201/b22852-4

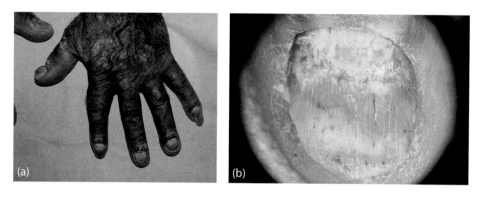

FIGURE 3.2 (a) Clinical and (b) onychoscopy of onycholysis due to nail psoriasis.

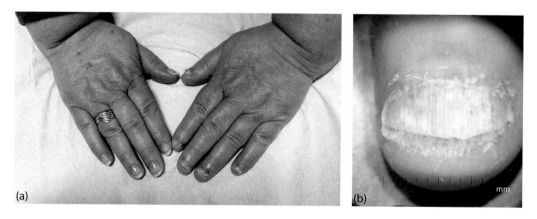

FIGURE 3.3 (a) Clinical and (b) onychoscopy of onycholysis due to onychomycosis.

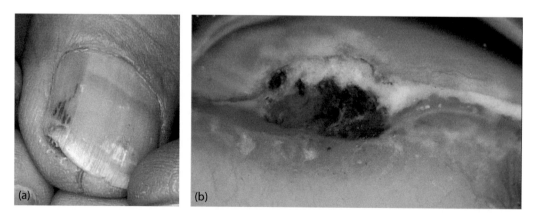

FIGURE 3.4 (a) Clinical and (b) onychoscopy of onycholysis due to subungual mass.

contact dermatitis may also cause onycholysis. Fungi are usually secondary colonizers as well as *Pseudomonas aeruginosa*. Drugs such as oxsoralen, tetracycline, minocycline, and naproxen can cause instead photo-onycholysis as the result of cutaneous photosensitization (**Figure 3.5**). Nail plate detachment usually appears after more than two weeks of exposure to the drug and often follows a photosensitivity reaction in the skin.

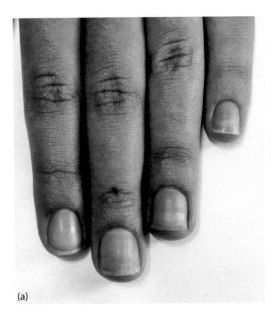
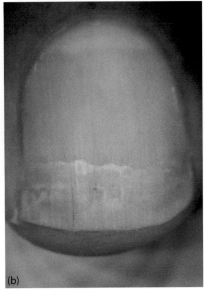

FIGURE 3.5   (a) Clinical and (b) onychoscopy of photo-onycholysis.

NAIL BED HYPERKERATOSIS

Subungual hyperkeratosis is a sign typical of a variety of nail diseases and for this reason, it is considered not specific for any disease in particular. It refers to the accumulation of scales under the nail plate, which sloughs off and which accumulates in this region. The nail bed is usually thicker than usual, and the nail plate is elevated from the nail bed due to the scales. The condition results from an excess of keratinocytes unable to be detached from the stratum corneum. In most nail conditions, hyperkeratosis slowly extends proximally. It can be localized or diffuse.

Common causes include onychomycosis, psoriasis, and chronic eczema (**Figures 3.6–3.8**). Other causes include congenital nail bed hyperplasia, pityriasis rubra pilaris, chronic nail bed trauma, aging, medications (venlafaxine, docetaxel, clofazimine), lichen planus and striatus, cutaneous sarcoidosis, pigmentary incontinence, Reiter's syndrome, discoid lupus erythematosus, Darier's disease, Norwegian scabies, reactive arthritis, Sézary syndrome,

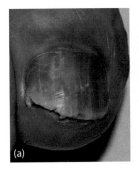
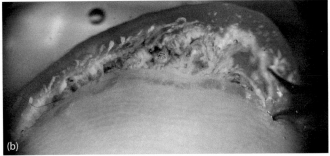

FIGURE 3.6   (a) Clinical and (b) onychoscopy of nail bed hyperkeratosis due to onychomycosis.

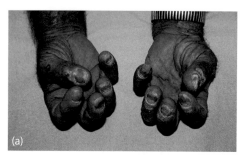
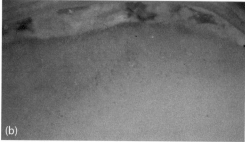

FIGURE 3.7   (a) Clinical and (b) onychoscopy of nail bed hyperkeratosis due to nail psoriasis.

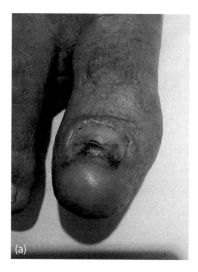
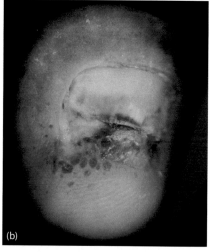

FIGURE 3.8   (a) Clinical and (b) onychoscopy of nail bed hyperkeratosis due to chronic eczema.

Langerhans cell histiocytosis, systemic malignancies, punctate keratoderma, and many other conditions. It is also found in some hyperkeratotic processes, such as warts, squamous cell carcinoma of the nail unit, and subungual epidermal inclusions (subungual onycholemal cysts) (**Figure 3.9**). In onychopapilloma, subungual hyperkeratosis is localized and

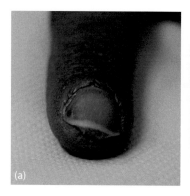
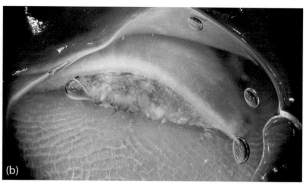

FIGURE 3.9   (a) Clinical and (b) onychoscopy of localized subungual hyperkeratosis due to squamous cell carcinoma.

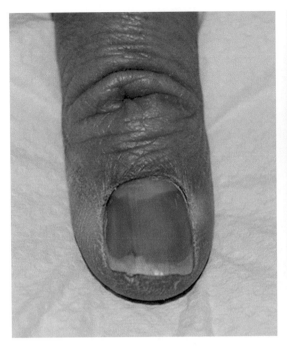
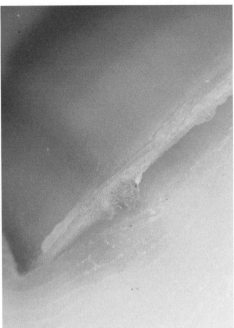

FIGURE 3.10   Onychoscopy of localized subungual hyperkeratosis due to onychopapilloma.

presents as a small lesion seen through the hyponychium (hyperkeratotic tip) (**Figure 3.10**), often associated with erythronychia in the nail plate.

"PUP TENT" SIGN

This is the characteristic finding of nail lichen planus. This alteration involves the nail bed and nail plate. Discrete red or purplish papules in the nail bed may uplift and split the overlapping plate lengthwise. The lateral edges slope downwards and give a "pup tent" appearance. Lichen planus as an isolated form of the nail bed is however rare, as nail bed involvement is usually seen in association with matrix disease (**Figure 3.11**).

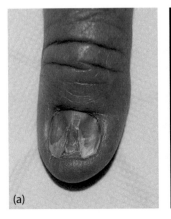
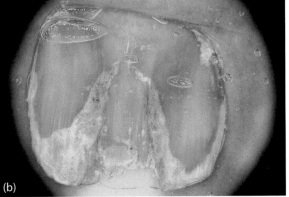

(a)

(b)

FIGURE 3.11   (a) Clinical and (b) onychoscopy of pup tent sign in nail bed lichen planus.

NAIL BED RETRACTION, DISAPPEARING NAIL BED, AND NAIL BED ATROPHY

As a consequence of inflammation, infections, and traumas, the nail bed may be exposed and as a consequence tend to shrink (**Figures 3.12** and **3.13**). That area becomes apparently cornified producing dermatoglyphics like the normal tip of a digit. This may explain why it is difficult to promote reattachment. It is generally assumed that the longer the disorder has been present, the less likely it is to resolve. The nail plate becomes short and thick and may also be permanently lost (**Figure 3.14**). Typical of lichen planus is nail bed atrophy due to the potential scarring outcome that this disease has. More in general these signs are associated with onychomycosis, postoperative period, trauma, retronychia, malalignment, onychophagia, and some congenital abnormalities.

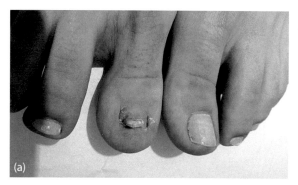
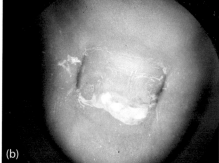

FIGURE 3.12   (a) Clinical and (b) onycoscopic pictures of trauma (disappearing nail bed).

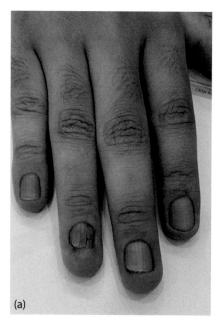
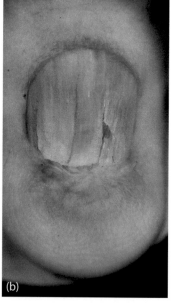

FIGURE 3.13   (a) Clinical and (b) onycoscopic pictures of lichen planus (atrophy).

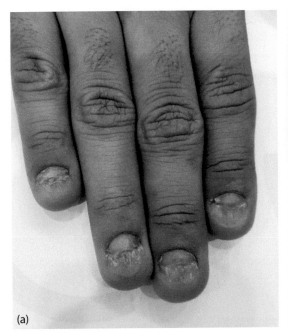
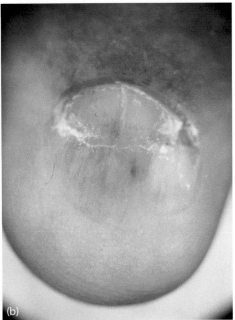

FIGURE 3.14   (a) Clinical and (b) onycoscopic pictures of lichen planus (nail plate short and atrophy of nail bed).

PTERYGIUM INVERSUM UNGUIS, VENTRAL PTERYGIUM

It is characterized by adherence of the distal nail bed to the ventral surface of the nail plate, resulting in obliteration of the distal sulcus at the hyponychium region (**Figure 3.15**). This condition can be congenital, idiopathic, secondary to systemic or other causes. It can be classified into three categories: congenital aberrant hyponychium, acquired irreversible form, and acquired reversible extended hyponychium. The acquired form may be associated with connective tissue diseases (systemic sclerosis, systemic lupus erythematosus), leprosy, onychophagia, allergic contact dermatitis, use of gel polish, and as a consequence

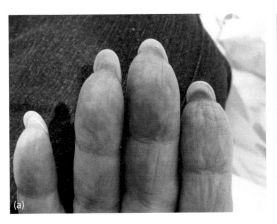
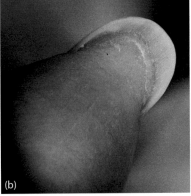

FIGURE 3.15   (a) Clinical and (b) onycoscopic pictures of pterygium inversum.

of allogeneic hematopoietic stem cell transplantation. The idiopathic form is often under-diagnosed and the exact origin remains speculative. The acquired form of the disease may be linked to abnormal distal circulation or exposure to certain chemical stimuli, which leads to matrix destruction, reactive hyperkeratosis, and pterygium formation.

CHROMONYCHIA

Melanonychia: A brown to black discoloration present in the nail bed can occur due to the presence of dematiaceous fungi responsible for fungal melanonychia, exogenous pigmentation (tobacco, silver nitrate), and post-inflammatory processes (nail lichen planus, onychotillomania, onychophagia, friction, tumors) (**Figures 3.16–3.19**).

In 2017, Perrin et al. confirmed the presence of melanocytes in the nail bed with immunohistochemical staining (HMB45, MITF, and Melan A antibodies). This study demonstrated a low density of melanocytes in the nail bed in contrast to the clearly higher density of melanocytes in the matrix. Therefore, melanonychia by melanocyte alteration can occur in the nail bed, being an uncommon process.

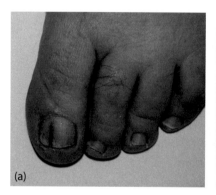
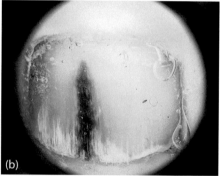

FIGURE 3.16   (a) Clinical and (b) onycoscopic pictures of fungal melanonychia.

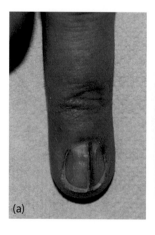
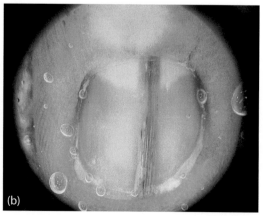

FIGURE 3.17   (a) Clinical and (b) onycoscopic pictures of melanonychia in pigmented tumors (onychopapilloma).

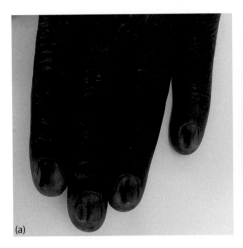
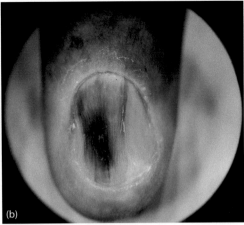

FIGURE 3.18 (a) Clinical and (b) onycoscopic pictures of melanonychia in post-inflammatory pigmentation of nail lichen planus.

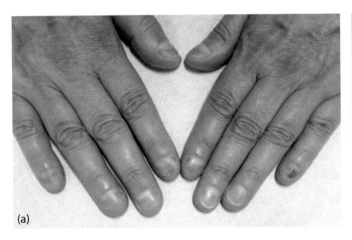
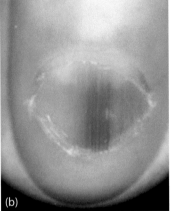

FIGURE 3.19 (a) Clinical and (b) onycoscopic pictures of melanonychia in onychofagia and onychotillomania.

Erythronychia: A reddish discoloration of the nail bed can occur due to local inflammatory changes such as psoriasis and lichen planus. Some tumors that occur in the nail bed, such as hemangiomas, glomus tumor, onychopapilloma, and some malignant tumors may also be responsible erythronychia as spots in the nail bed or longitudinal streaks (**Figures 3.20–3.23**).

Leukonychia: The nail bed appears paler than usual in three different situations described below. Leukonychia affecting the nail bed is a form of apparent leukonychia that fades with pressure on the nail plate because pressure results in temporary reduction of nail bed edema and then better visibility of nail bed vessels. Apparent partial/total leukonychia can be seen rather frequently and are often medical-relevant leukonychias.

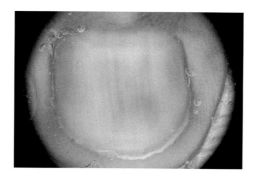

FIGURE 3.20 Clinical picture of nail bed erythronychia due to glomus tumor.

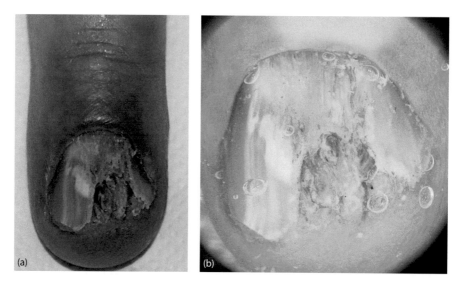

FIGURE 3.21 (a) Clinical and (b) onycoscopic pictures of nail bed erythronychia due to squamous cell carcinoma.

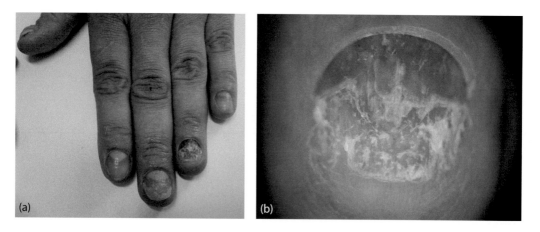

FIGURE 3.22 (a) Clinical and (b) onycoscopic pictures of nail bed erythronychia due to nail psoriasis.

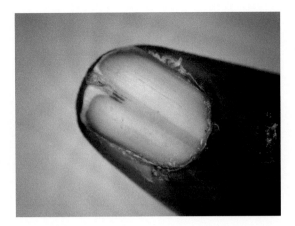

FIGURE 3.23   Onycoscopic picture of nail bed erythronychia due to onychopapilloma.

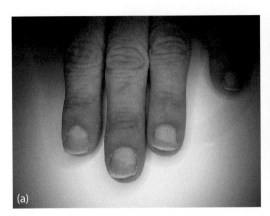
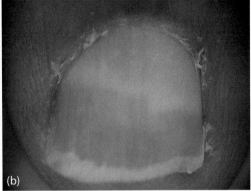

FIGURE 3.24   (a) Clinical and (b) onycoscopic pictures of nail bed leukonychia in half-and-half nails.

1. *Half-and-half nails*: These also known as Lindsay's nails, are characterized by a sharply demarcated red, pink, or brown discoloration of 20%–60% of the distal nail bed, leading to two-colored nails with a transverse border. Half-and-half nails are detected in approximately in 10%–30% of patients with chronic renal disease (uremic patients and patients on hemodialysis) (**Figure 3.24**).

2. *Terry's nails*: These are characterized by a bilaterally symmetrical white nail bed of the fingernails with a distal band, 1–2 mm in length, that had a normal pink or erythematous color. It has been supposed that the distal erythematous crescent probably is a prominent onychodermal band. Histological studies of the nail bed have shown vascular changes (telangiectasias) in the bands. While being promoted as one of the most reliable physical signs of cirrhosis and early sign of autoimmune hepatitis, Terry's nails can also be an indication of chronic renal failure, congestive heart failure, hematologic disease, adult-onset diabetes mellitus, but also occur with normal aging (**Figure 3.25**).

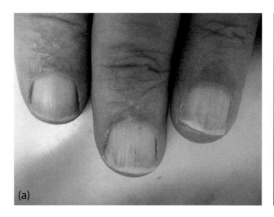
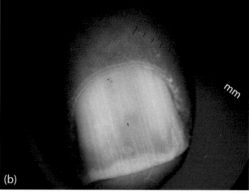

FIGURE 3.25   (a) Clinical and (b) onycoscopic pictures of nail bed leukonychia in Terry's nails.

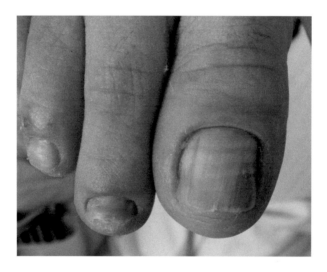

FIGURE 3.26   Clinical picture of nail bed leukonychia in Muehrcke's nails.

3. *Muehrcke's nails* present with narrow transverse white bands. They are parallel to the lunula, separated from each other by pink strips. Initially described in patients with severe and longstanding hypoalbuminemia, nowadays they are considered indicative of a range of systemic pathologies without hypoalbuminemia, including kidney disease, rheumatoid arthritis, and heart transplant. Cytotoxic drugs and retinoids can also produce Muehrcke bands (**Figure 3.26**).

SPLINTER HEMORRHAGES

They are a frequent and nonspecific clinical finding described in various nail disorders, trauma-induced, drug-induced, and even idiopathic (**Figures 3.27–3.29**). They occur due to extravasation of blood following local vasodilation or minor local trauma. Initially, they occur as reddish microdots, but with continued growth of the nail plate, they become elongated and darker. They are asymptomatic, tiny, linear, reddish-brown to black, longitudinal streaks 1–3 mm long that appear under the nail plate.

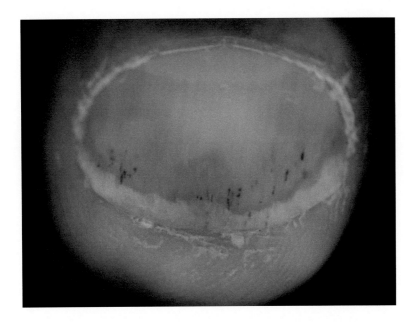

FIGURE 3.27   Onycoscopic pictures of splinter hemorrhages in nail psoriasis.

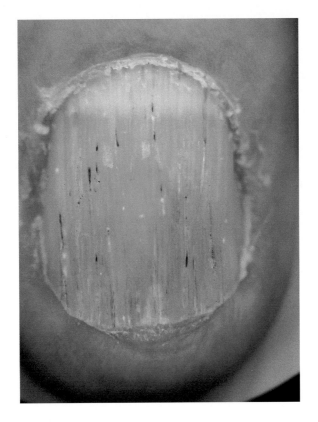

FIGURE 3.28   Onycoscopic pictures of splinter hemorrhages in nail lichen planus.

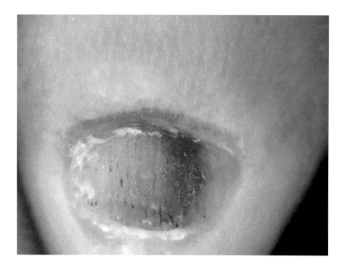

FIGURE 3.29 Onycoscopic pictures of splinter hemorrhages of fifth toe trauma.

SUGGESTED READINGS

Baran R, Juhlin L. Drug-induced photo-onycholysis. Three subtypes identified in a study of 15 cases. *J Am Acad Dermatol.* 1987;17(6):1012–6.

Daniel CR 3rd, Iorizzo M, Piraccini BM, Tosti A. Simple onycholysis. *Cutis.* 2011;87(5):226–8.

Daniel CR III, Meir B, Avner S. An update on the disappearing nail bed. *Skin Appendage Disord.* 2017;3(1):15–17.

Finch J, Arenas R, Baran R. Fungal melanonychia. *J Am Acad Dermatol.* 2012;66(5):830–41.

Haber R, Khoury R, Kechichian E, Tomb R. Splinter hemorrhages of the nails: a systematic review of clinical features and associated conditions. *International Journal of Dermatology.* 2016;55(12):1304–1310.

Mello C, Chiacchio N. Ruin appearance in nail free margin dermoscopy - a diagnostic clue for onychomycosis. *Surg Cosmet Dermatol.* 2019;11(3):232–3.

Naveen KN. Pup tent sign. *Indian Dermatol Online J.* 2014;5(4):552–3.

Perrin C, Michiels JF, Boyer J, Ambrosetti D. Melanocytes pattern in the normal nail, with special reference to nail bed melanocytes. *Am J Dermatopathol.* 2018;40(3):180–4.

Zaias N, Escovar SX, Zaiac MN. Finger and toenail onycholysis. *J Eur Acad Dermatol Venereol.* 2015;29(5):848–53.

CHAPTER 4

Nail Plate Signs

THIS CHAPTER DEALS WITH NAIL PLATE SIGNS AND CHANGES IN ITS CONFIGURATION that are not the result of alterations in the nail matrix but are due to other causes.

CHANGES IN THE TRANSVERSE CURVATURE

Pincer nails are characterized by transverse overcurvature of the nail plate that increases along the longitudinal axis of the nail towards the tip. The curvature is reduced proximally and greater distally. At the tip of the digit, the nail plate pinches the soft periungual tissues constricting, with pain, the underlying nail bed. It can occur in both toenails and fingernails. However, the toenails are most commonly affected. It could have a hereditary or acquired origin. This deformity may cause cosmetic problems as well as pain and discomfort when walking or wearing shoes. Osteophytes are often present in the distal part of the last phalanx contributing to pain perception. The associations with osteoarthritis, onychomycosis, or use of ß-blockers have been reported (**Figure 4.1**).

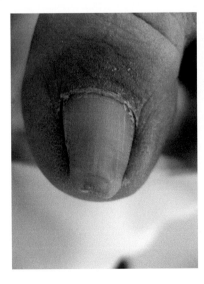 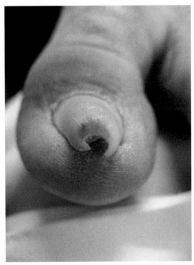

FIGURE 4.1   Clinical pictures of pincer nail.

DOI: 10.1201/b22852-5

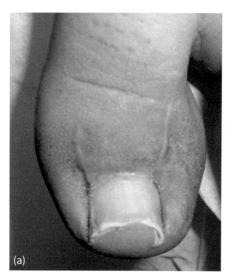
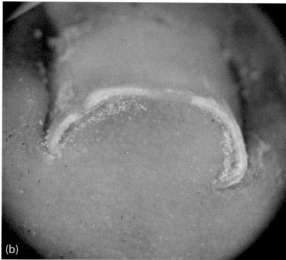

FIGURE 4.2 (a) Clinical and (b) onychoscopy pictures of tile-shaped nail.

Tile-shaped nails are characterized by an even greater increase in the transverse curvature along the longitudinal axis of the nail plate. The curvature maintains the same proportion in the proximal and distal regions (**Figure 4.2**).

Plicated nails are characterized by a nail plate surface almost flat. One or both lateral margins are angled and can press into the lateral nail grooves producing sometimes granulation tissue, mimicking an ingrown nail (**Figure 4.3**).

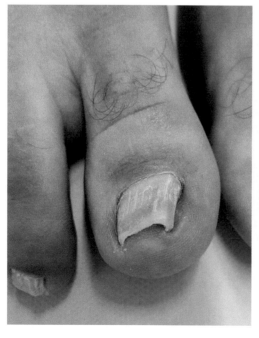
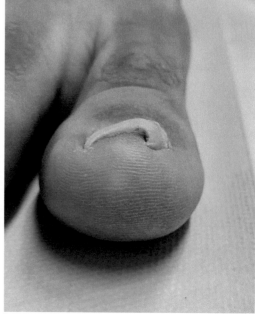

FIGURE 4.3 Clinical pictures of plicated nail.

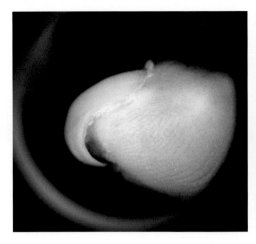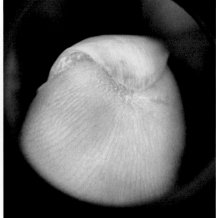

FIGURE 4.4 Onychoscopy of parrot beak nail.

CHANGES IN THE LONGITUDINAL CURVATURE

Parrot beak nails are characterized by a peculiar symmetrical longitudinal overcurvature of the free margin that resembles a parrot's beak. It is typically an incidental finding, after fingertip injury or amputation due to bone loss, loss of nail bed support, and scarring contracture. However, it can also occur congenitally in patients with skeletal abnormalities, associated with systemic sclerosis, or chronic crack-cocaine abuse involving ischemia processes (**Figure 4.4**).

Claw nail describes a morphological alteration of the nail plate characterized by a dorsal curvature with a concave upper surface. It is often associated with the development of local calluses. This condition predominates in one or more toenails, in women who wear high heels and narrow shoes. Claw-like birth defects have also been reported.

Overcurvature of the fourth toenail is a rare disorder, often bilateral without other anomalies of the extremities, usually asymptomatic. The cause is still unknown, but it is thought to be due to shortening of the distal phalanx and hypoplasia of soft tissue of the fourth toe (**Figure 4.5**).

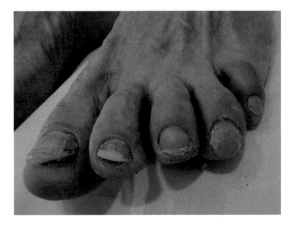

FIGURE 4.5 Clinical picture of overcurvature of the fourth toenail.

CHANGES IN LONGITUDINAL AND TRANSVERSE CURVATURE

Clubbing also known as hippocratic nails, watch-glass nails, and drumstick fingers. It is characterized by increased transverse and longitudinal nail curvature with hypertrophy of the soft-tissue components of the digit pulp (**Figure 4.6**). The most promising hypothesis proposed to explain the pathophysiology holds that megakaryocytes or platelet clusters, housed in the peripheral vasculature of the fingers, release platelet-derived growth factor and lead to increased vascularity, permeability, and connective tissue changes.

There are three forms of geometric assessment that can be performed to verify if we are dealing with clubbing. *Lovibond's angle* is found at the junction between the nail plate and the proximal nail fold and is normally less than 160°. This is altered to over 180° in clubbing. *Curth's angle* at the distal interphalangeal joint is normally about 180°. This is diminished to less than 160° in clubbing. *Schamroth's window* is seen when the dorsal aspects of two fingers from opposite hands are opposed, revealing a window of light, bordered laterally by the Lovibond angle. As this angle is obliterated in clubbing, the window closes. Clubbing is associated with a variety of clinical conditions including pulmonary diseases, liver cirrhosis, cyanotic congenital heart disease, malignancies, and underlying suppurative conditions or it can occur as an isolated finding.

Koilonychia presents with a flat nail plate and is spoon-shaped due to upward eversion of its lateral edges. Although koilonychia, which is frequent and physiological in the toenails of children, has been reported in association with a large number of systemic conditions, the only disorder that should be routinely ruled out in adults is severe iron-deficiency anemia. Familial forms are also known (**Figure 4.7**).

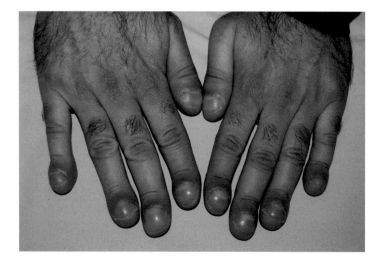

FIGURE 4.6   Clinical picture of clubbing.

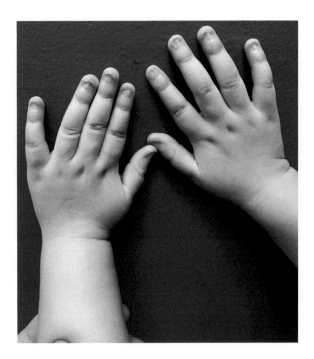

FIGURE 4.7   Clinical picture of koilonychia of finger nail.

CHANGES IN THE SURFACE

Washboard nails are an uncommon nail disorder that usually affects the thumbnails. The condition is asymptomatic and most often symmetrical. It is characterized by a median longitudinal groove with smaller transverse ridges, radiating from this paramedian canal (**Figure 4.8**). The self-inflicted nail trauma involving manipulation of

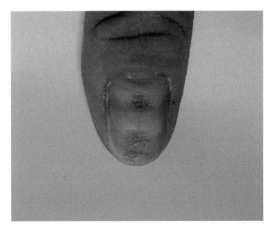
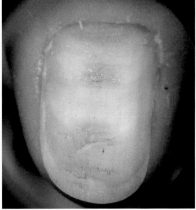

FIGURE 4.8   Median canaliform nail dystrophy in wash board nail.

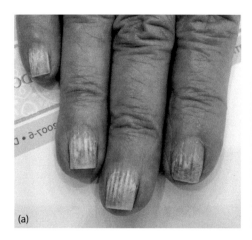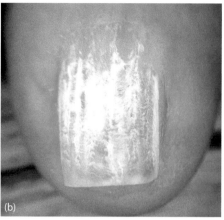

(a)   (b)

FIGURE 4.9   (a) Clinical and (b) onychoscopy of superficial granulation of keratin.

the cuticle and proximal nail fold as part of tic habit has been identified as a common cause.

Superficial granulation of keratin is a brittleness confined to the nail plate surface. Nail polish abuse damage the superficial layers of the nail plate and tight attachment of onychocytes so the upper layers of the plate start to scale. Keratin degranulation is a type of pseudoleukonychia and should not be confused with superficial white onychomycosis (**Figures 4.9** and **4.10**).

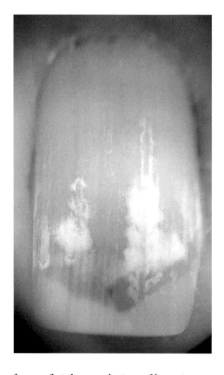

FIGURE 4.10   Onychoscopy of superficial granulation of keratin.

Elkonyxis is a condition that shows irregular defects in the dorsal nail plate. It is clinically characterized by a punched-out lesion at the lunula that progressively moves distally with the nail growth. This has been described secondary to syphilis, psoriasis, Reiter's syndrome, and after trauma. It has also been reported in association with retinoid therapy (**Figures 4.11** and **4.12**).

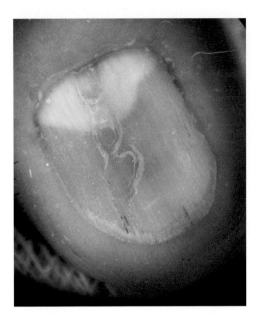

FIGURE 4.11   Onychoscopy of elkonyxis.

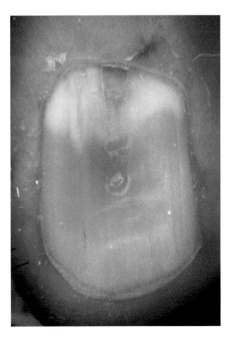

FIGURE 4.12   Onychoscopy of elkonyxis.

SUGGESTED READINGS

Allegue F, González-Vilas D, Zulaica A. Elconixis por isotretinoína. *Actas Dermo-Sifiliográficas.* 2017;108(2):166–167.

Chen SX, Cohen PR. Parrot beak nails revisited: case series and comprehensive review. *Dermatol Ther.* 2017;8(1):147–155.

Cohen PR, Milewicz DM. Dolichonychia in women with Marfan syndrome. *South Med J.* 2004;97(4):354–8.

Hirata Y, Shiiya C, Miyamoto J, Saito M. Congenital curved nail of the fourth toe: report of three cases and review of the literature. *J Dermatol.* 2022;49(9):925–927.

Lee JI, Lee YB, Oh ST, Park HJ, Cho BK. A clinical study of 35 cases of pincer nails. *Ann Dermatol.* 2011;23(4):417.

Pathania V. Median canaliform dystrophy of Heller occurring on thumb and great toe nails. *Med J Armed Forces India.* 2016;72(2):178–179.

Sarkar M, Mahesh D, Madabhavi I. Digital clubbing. *Lung India.* 2012;29(4):354. doi:10.4103/0970-2113.102824

CHAPTER 5

Periungual Signs

DORSAL PTERYGIUM

Dorsal pterygium or pterygium unguis results from a focal destruction of the nail matrix with subsequent scar formation. Because a nail plate is not formed at the affected site, the proximal nail fold epithelium attaches directly to the nail bed epithelium and both grow distally together to produce a wing-shaped deformity. Pterygium unguis usually affects the fingers and rarely the toes. It is the hallmark of severe lichen planus, although it is not specific. It can occur after trauma. Multiple pterium in the same nails have been described (**Figure 5.1** and **5.2**).

The pathogenesis of pterygium is complex and poorly understood. Some authors have suggested that it is the result of lymphocyte-mediated destruction of the nail unit. More recently, it has been reported that **pterygium** results from a violent inflammation resulting in a fibrotic process that leads to the fusion of the nail fold with the nail bed. This fibrosis prevents the normal growth of the nail plate, which then appears divided or completely destroyed.

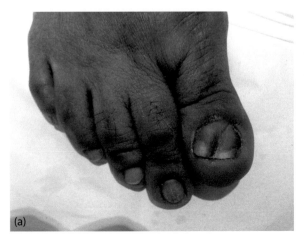
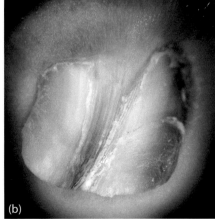

FIGURE 5.1   (a) Clinical and (b) onychoscopy pictures of dorsal pterygium.

DOI: 10.1201/b22852-6

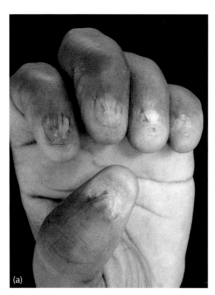
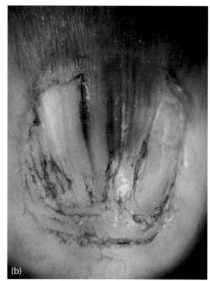

FIGURE 5.2 (a) Clinical and (b) onychoscopy pictures of dorsal pterygium.

CUTICLE ABNORMALITIES

The cuticle, the horny layer of the epidermis of the proximal nail fold, may be altered. Thickened, hyperkeratotic, and irregular (ragged) cuticles have been reported, especially in dermatomyositis. It is common that in chronic inflammatory conditions as paronychia the cuticle disappears. The habit of pushing the cuticle away is a cultural habit in women who like to decorate their nails, but it should be discouraged (**Figures 5.3–5.5**).

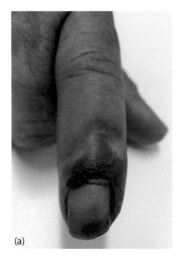
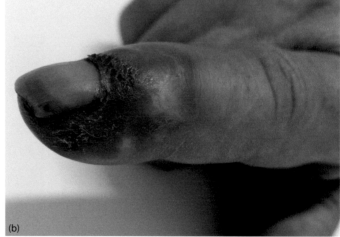

FIGURE 5.3 (a) Clinical and (b) onychoscopy pictures of acute paronychia.

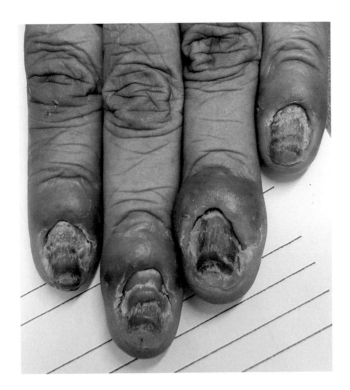

FIGURE 5.4   Clinical picture of chronic paronychia.

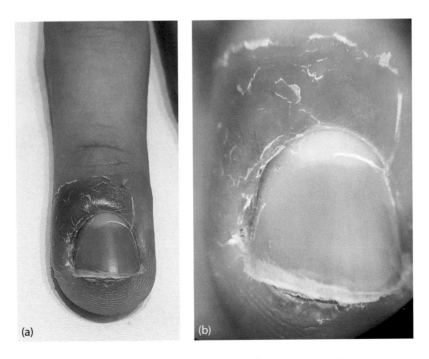

(a)

(b)

FIGURE 5.5   (a) Clinical and (b) onychoscopy pictures of acute paronychia.

VASCULAR CHANGES OF THE NAIL FOLDS

Pyogenic granuloma is an acquired benign vascular lesion that can occur in the proximal or lateral nail folds and presents as a painful, smooth, sessile or pedunculated, red, rapidly growing, and often bleeding lesion. One or more lesions can be observed in one or more fingers. They are common after trauma. They can also be drug-induced (retinoids, chemotherapy agents). Other causes may be peripheral nerve injury, infection, and pregnancy (**Figures 5.6–5.8**).

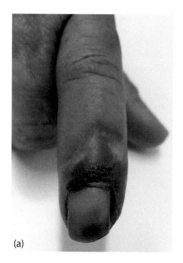
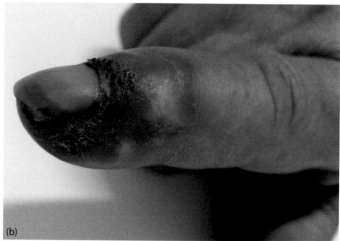

(a) (b)

FIGURE 5.6   (a) Clinical and (b) onychoscopy pictures of dorsal pterygium.

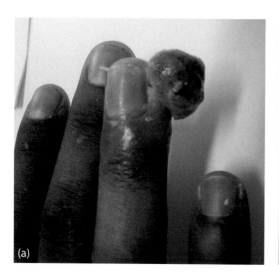
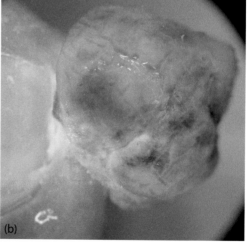

(a) (b)

FIGURE 5.7   (a) Clinical and (b) onychoscopy pictures of lateral pyogenic granuloma.

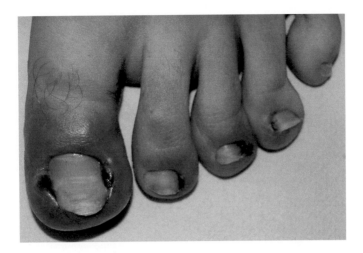

FIGURE 5.8   Clinical picture of mutiple periungual pygenic granuloma due to erlotinib.

Periungual telangiectasia can be associated with collagen vascular diseases where relative tissue anoxia may cause the appearance of telangiectasias, especially in acral areas. This is especially true for systemic lupus erythematosus and progressive systemic sclerosis. Circulating cryoglobulins may also lead to acral telangiectasias (**Figure 5.9**).

Changes in microcirculation of the nail fold are typical of connective tissue diseases and diagnostic patterns have been described by capillaroscopy and more recently by dermoscopy.

1. The scleroderma pattern presents with micro-hemorrhages, disorganization of the capillary architecture (irregular distribution, orientation, and morphology), avascular areas and thickened cuticle. It is possible to identify three different stages: early (limited number of giant capillaries, rare microhaemorrhages), active (numerous giant capillaries, frequent microhaemorrhages, moderate reduction of capillary density), and late (marked loss of capillaries with evident extensive avascular areas and ramified or

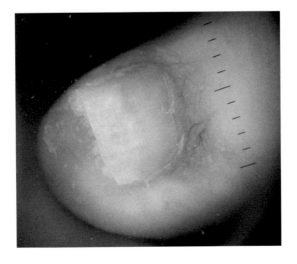

FIGURE 5.9   Onychoscopy of acral telangiectasias.

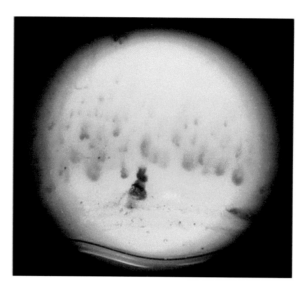

FIGURE 5.10   Capillaroscopy of systemic sclerosis.

bushy neoangiogenesis). Some of these capillary alterations may precede the symptoms of connective tissue diseases and may herald disease before clinical manifestation (**Figure 5.10**).

2. The dermatomyositis pattern presents with tortuous and dilated capillaries, giant capillaries, and neo-angiogenesis. Arborization and bushy capillaries are typical of the end stages. The typical alterations are present in 75% of patients with dermatomyositis (**Figure 5.11**).

3. The lupus pattern is less specific with enlarged tortuous capillaries and normal capillary density. The capillary pattern is normal in most patients, but in 30% the most frequent changes are nonspecific, such as increased tortuous loops, sometimes with serpiginous appearance, stretched loops and oddly shaped, greater visibility of the venous plexus sub-papillary that has an increased diameter (**Figure 5.12**).

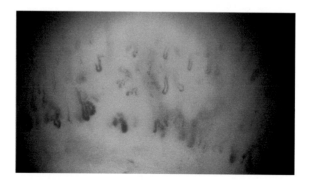

FIGURE 5.11   Capillaroscopy of dermatomyositis.

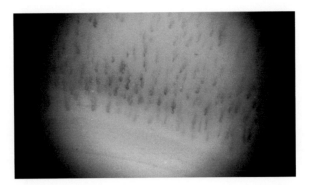

FIGURE 5.12   Capillaroscopy of LES.

SUGGESTED READINGS

Alessandrini A, Bruni F, Starace M, Piraccini BM. Periungual pyogenic granuloma: the importance of the medical history. *Skin Appendage Disord.* 2016;1(4):175–8.

Chang P, Argueta TG, Cohen SEN, et al. Manifestaciones del aparato ungueal en las enfermedades del colágeno: reporte de 43 casos. *Dermatol Cosmét Méd Quir.* 2016;14(4):270–80.

Grover C, Jakhar D, Mishra A, Singal A. Nail-fold capillaroscopy for the dermatologists. *Indian J Dermatol Venereol Leprol.* 2022;88(3):300–3–12.

Koga H, Saida T, Uhara H. Key point in dermoscopic differentiation between early nail apparatus melanoma and benign longitudinal melanonychia. *J Dermatol.* 2011;38(1):45–52.

Ronger S, Touzet S, Ligeron C, et al. Dermoscopic examination of nail pigmentation. *Arch Dermatol.* 2002;138(10):1327–33.

II

Nail Disorders

CHAPTER 6

Acute Paronychia

A CUTE PARONYCHIA IS AN ACUTE INFLAMMATORY PROCESS AFFECTING THE NAIL FOLDS with less than six weeks of evolution. Despite the numerous causes, trauma resulting from aggressive manicure, onychophagia/cuticle picking, or penetration of foreign bodies are the most common triggering factors. The broken-down cuticle, the physical barrier between the nail plate and the nail folds, allows the infiltration of infectious organisms, allergens, or irritants. Other causes such as pemphigus vulgaris, pustular psoriasis, and drugs (chemotherapeutic agents, systemic retinoids, and antiretroviral drugs) are also reported as causative agents. The lesion starts 2–5 days after the causal factor with erythema, edema and pain, and possible purulent discharge. Other infectious agents (herpes simplex, fungi and syphilis for example) can mimic acute paronychia due to bacteria – this is why culture test should be mandatory before prescribing treatment (**Figures 6.1–6.3**).

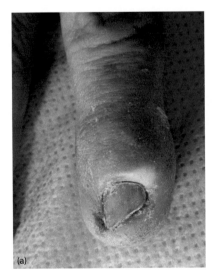
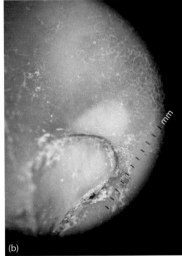

FIGURE 6.1   (a) Acute paronychia with swelling of the proximal nail fold. A collection of pus is clearly visible in the periungual area. (b) Dermoscopy view allows a better visualization of the periungual erythema with scales, associated with whitish area that represents the purulent process.

DOI: 10.1201/b22852-8

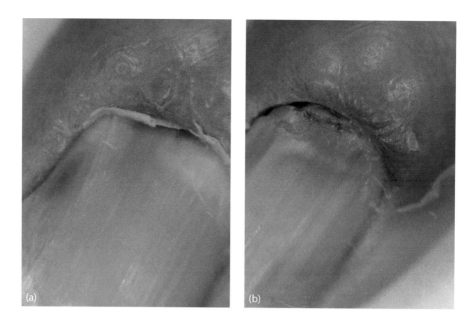

FIGURE 6.2 Dermoscopy view of acute paronychia (a) responsible for onychomadesis (b). Note in panel (a) the collection of pus behind the plate and the discharge (b) once the plate is detached from bed.

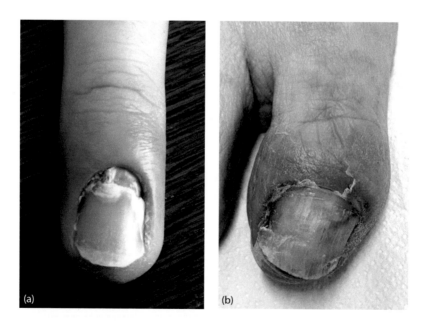

FIGURE 6.3 (a) Acute paronychia without bacterial infection. (b) Acute paronychia associated with onychomycosis due to molds.

SUGGESTED READING

Rigopoulos D, Larios G, Gregoriou S, Alevizos A. Acute and chronic paronychia. *Am Fam Physician* 2008;77:339–346.

CHAPTER 7

Chronic Paronychia

CHRONIC PARONYCHIA IS CONSIDERED AN INFLAMMATORY DISEASE LASTING MORE than six weeks, involving one or more nail folds (lateral and proximal). It is more common in workers with frequent contact with soap and water, or in those who have the habit of removing the cuticles. A persistent inflammatory reaction that impairs nail fold keratinization and prevents the formation of a new cuticle maintains the condition over time. Cuticle loss creates a space between the nail plate and the proximal fold that allows entry of irritants, allergens, and microorganisms. The chronicity of the inflammation usually leads to a dystrophic nail plate. Swelling of proximal nail fold, cuticle absence, and nail plate dystrophy with transversal grooves are typical of this condition.

In patients with chronic mucocutaneous candidiasis and HIV infection, proximal nail fold inflammation is usually associated with proximal onycholysis or onychomycosis due to *Candida* (**Figures 7.1** and **7.2**).

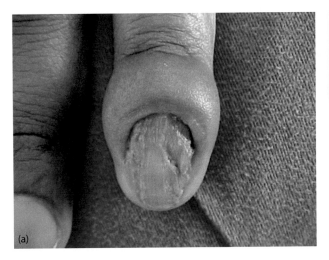 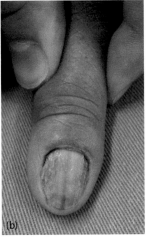

(a) (b)

FIGURE 7.1 Clinical aspect of a chronic paronychia (a) revealing the absence of the cuticle, swelling of the proximal nail fold, opening of the cuticle sac zone, and nail plate alteration (b) as well as longitudinal melanonychia (melanocytic activation).

DOI: 10.1201/b22852-9

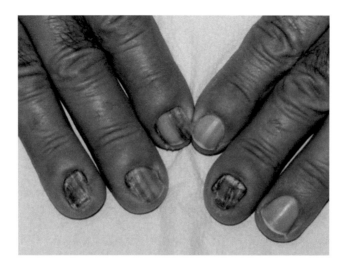

FIGURE 7.2 Chronic paronychia of multiple fingernails with longitudinal bands of melanocytic activation.

SUGGESTED READING

Daniel CR III, Daniel MP, Daniel CM, et al. Chronic paronychia and onycholysis: a 13 year experience. *Cutis* 1996;58:397–401.

CHAPTER 8

Periungual Eczema

I T MAY OCCUR ASSOCIATED WITH ANY TYPE OF ECZEMA—MAINLY ATOPIC DERMATITIS, allergic or irritant contact dermatitis. A good anamnesis is mandatory for the diagnosis. The history of exposure to an allergen, such as dichromate, nickel, cobalt, fragrance mix, epoxy resin, thiuram mix, paraphenylenediamine, and formaldehyde, is very common in cases of allergic contact dermatitis. Alkalis, acids, soaps, solvents, and abrasives are often reported in cases of irritant contact dermatitis. Clinical features depend on the area of nail unit involved. When the inflammatory infiltrate involves the nail matrix, nail pitting, trachyonichia, longitudinal ridges, transverse grooves, Beau's lines, and onycomadesis are often observed. Chromonychia, onycholysis, and splinter hemorrhages are due to bed involvement, while paronychia, pulpitis, fissuring, erythema, scales, and loss of cuticles are typical of periungual tissues involvement (**Figures 8.1** and **8.2**).

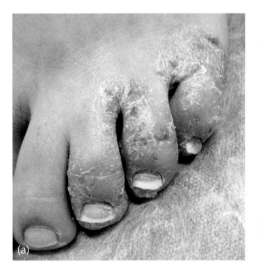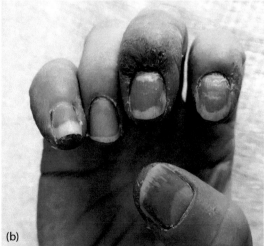

FIGURE 8.1   (a) Periungual eczema showing Beau's lines, (b) onychomadesis, onycholysis, and subungual scales.

DOI: 10.1201/b22852-10

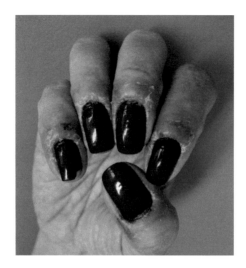

FIGURE 8.2   Clinical aspect of periungual eczema due to nail polish.

SUGGESTED READINGS

Savitha AS, Shashikumar BM. Nail changes in eczemas and miscellaneous disorders. In Grover C, Relhan V, Nanda S, et al., eds. *Textbook of Onychology*. New Delhi, Evangel 2021:217–219.

Tyagi M, Singal A. Nail cosmetics: What a dermatologist should know! *Indian J Dermatol Venereol Leprol*. 2023 May 29:1–8.

CHAPTER 9

Herpes Simplex

IT IS CAUSED BY HERPES SIMPLEX VIRUS TYPE 1 AND 2, AND IT IS MORE FREQUENT IN THE index finger of women and children. The lesion starts with typical vesicles on erythematous and edematous base, extremely painful. After some days, vesicles often coalesce into bullae, and fluid becomes turbid, purulent, or even hemorrhagic. Then crusts appear and heal completely in 15 days on average. Diagnosis should be confirmed by Tzanck smear or culture or polymerase chain reaction or serum analysis because the clinical picture is very similar to a bacterial infection. The main point in favor of dermoscopy is the better view of the vesicles that, sometimes, could not be seen with the naked eye (**Figures 9.1** and **9.2**).

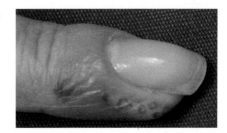

FIGURE 9.1 Periungual herpes simplex with erythema, edema, and vesicles.

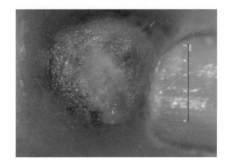

FIGURE 9.2 Periungual herpes simplex—dermoscopy of a big vesicle.

SUGGESTED READING

Iorizzo M, Pasch MC. Bacterial and viral infections of the nail unit. *Dermatol Clin* 2021;39: 245–253.

DOI: 10.1201/b22852-11

CHAPTER 10

Onychomycosis

ONYCHOMYCOSIS MEANS FUNGAL INFECTION OF THE NAIL UNIT. Dermatophytes are responsible for the majority of cases, others are due to molds and yeasts. Distal and lateral subungual onychomycosis due to *Trichophyton rubrum* is the most common type. Fungi enter the nail unit through the hyponychium and infect the area beneath the nail plate, moving proximally and showing the following dermoscopic patterns: jagged proximal margin of the onycholytic area, sharp structures (spikes), and white-yellow longitudinal striae directed to the proximal fold (which corresponds to the outbreak of fungal invasion). The "ruin appearance" is instead the dermatoscopic pattern of subungual hyperkeratosis that develops owing to the build-up of dermal debris from fungal invasion (**Figures 10.1–10.4**). Dermatophytoma is an aggregation of hyphae and scales in the subungual region that can be better appreciated by dermoscopy as yellow-orange patch, connected to the distal edge of the nail plate by a thin narrow channel (**Figure 10.5**). Fungi can also produce dark pigment, rarely in bands and more at random (fungal melanonychia). Together with dermatophytoma it is a sign of treatment resisitance.

Proximal subungual onychomycosis usually produces a white/yellowish area in the lunula area. At the same time, the remaining nail plate is unaffected as the fungi reach the ventral portion of the nail plate through the undersurface of the proximal nail fold (**Figure 10.6**).

White superficial onychomycosis can also be observed, and it is mostly due to *Trichophyton mentagrophytes*. Small white spots on the dorsal surface of the nail plate correspond *to* fungal colonies. Involvement of the whole thickness of the nail plate is also possible (deep variant) (**Figures 10.7** and **10.8**).

Mold onychomycosis can often be clinically suspected due to the presence of periungual inflammation. *Candida* may also affect nails. In healthy newborns, it resolves in a few months and has been associated with contamination during delivery and generally due to vaginal candidiasis of the mother. In older children and adults, it is observed in the presence of immunological defects. Chronic mucocutaneous candidiasis is characterized by chronic *Candida* infection of the skin, the mucous membranes, and the nails. In this condition, *Candida* invades the nails producing total onychomycosis. The affected nails are thickened, crumbly, and yellow-brown in color with more or less severe paronychia.

DOI: 10.1201/b22852-12

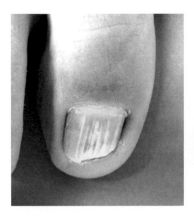
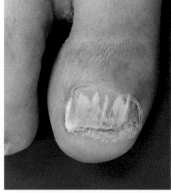

FIGURE 10.1   Distal subungual onychomycosis white-yellow longitudinal striae along the nail plate.

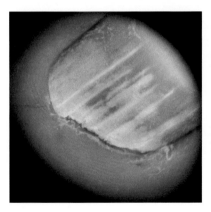
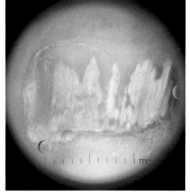

FIGURE 10.2   Dermoscopy allows a better visualization of the proximal progression of fungi along the horny layer of the nail plate.

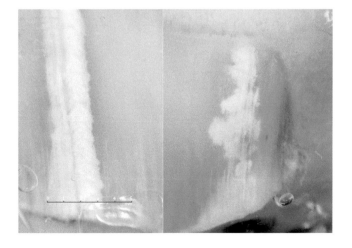

FIGURE 10.3   Yellow/white spikes or round areas (fluffy shadows) of infection.

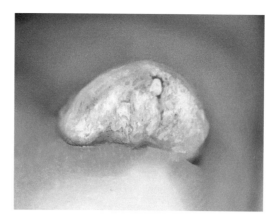

FIGURE 10.4   Ruin like appearance and scales typical of fungal infection.

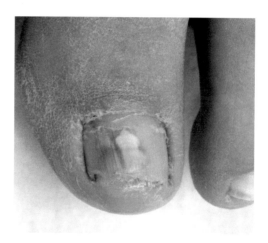

FIGURE 10.5   Dermatophytoma.

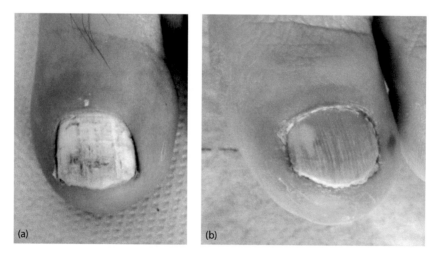

FIGURE 10.6   Deep variant. (a) Clinically—white spots on the dorsal surface of the nail plate are observed. (b) Small white opaque and friable patches.

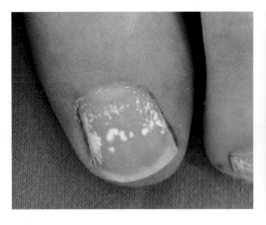 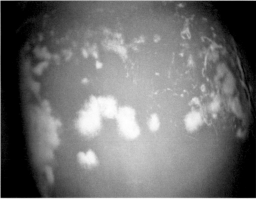

FIGURE 10.7   (a) Superficial variant. (b) Proximal subungual onychomycosis.

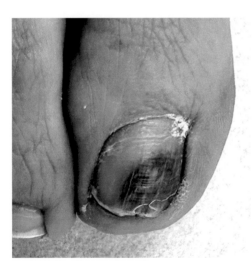 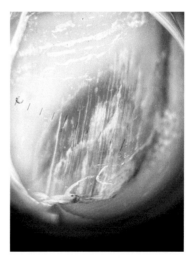

FIGURE 10.8   Pigmented onychomycosis—the yellow longitudinal streak helps in the differential diagnosis of *Pseudomonas aeruginosa* infection.

SUGGESTED READINGS

Lipner SR, Scher RK. Onychomycosis: clinical overview and diagnosis. *J Am Acad Dermatol* 2019;80:835–851.

Ohn J, et al. Dermoscopic patterns of fungal melanonychia: A comparative study with other causes of melanonychia. *J Am Acad Dermatol* 2017;76:488–493

Piraccini BM, Balestri R, Starace M, Rech G. Nail digital dermoscopy (onychoscopy) in the diagnosis of onychomycosis. *J Eur Acad Dermatol Venereol* 2013;27:509–513.

CHAPTER 11

Nail Psoriasis

THE CLINICAL FINDINGS OF NAIL PSORIASIS DEPEND ON THE AREA OF THE NAIL apparatus affected by the inflammatory infiltrate—nail matrix or nail bed or periungual tissues. When the matrix is involved, the plate shows irregular pitting, thickening, and crumbling, and more rarely a red lunula is visible through the proximal portion. When the bed is involved, onycholysis, subungual keratosis, and splinter hemorrhages are typical signs. When the periungual tissues are involved, it is common to see paronychia with inflammation and scales. All these signs could present isolated or freely combined in the same patient and even in the same nail. Some of them are however not unique to psoriasis, and for this reason, the diagnosis is often delayed. Onychomycosis is frequently associated with further delaying of the diagnosis. Due to the relation that nail psoriasis has with psoriatic arthritis, great attention should be addressed to the nail signs that might reveal a possible joint involvement in order to early refer patients to a rheumatologist and even contributing to the prevention of arthritis. Pitting and, above all, onycholysis seem to occur more often in patients with arthritis compared to those without.

The pits of psoriasis are irregularly distributed, are large and deep (which differ from the ones of alopecia areata that are smaller, regular in shape, size, and distribution), and may be associated with proximal diffuse scale. Crumbling, a sign of severe nail matrix psoriasis, presents as proximal nail plate irregularities.

Nail bed signs are better visualized with dermoscopy and when an ultrasound gel is applied as an interface solution, it is possible to see the erythematous proximal border of onycholysis with the typical slightly dented margin. This margin can only be seen with dermoscopy and is a unique feature of nail psoriasis allowing the differential diagnosis with other causes of onycholysis, such as those caused by trauma or fungus.

Finally, dermoscopy of the hyponychium can reveal capillaries dilated, tortuous, and elongated. These findings are easier to see at 40× magnifications, although they can be appreciated with a handheld dermatoscope as regular red dots (**Figures 11.1–11.6**).

DOI: 10.1201/b22852-13

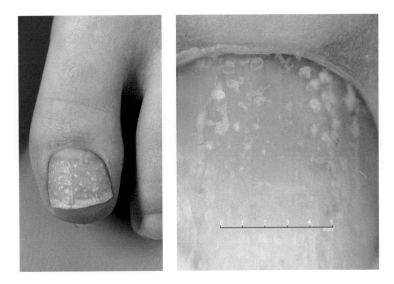

FIGURE 11.1   Pitting—irregularly distributed, large, and deep.

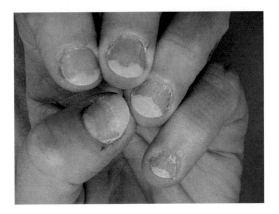

FIGURE 11.2   Onycholysis affecting all digits.

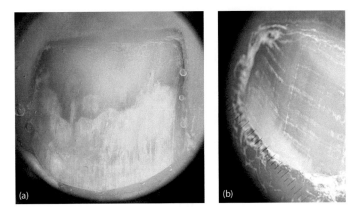

FIGURE 11.3   Dented onycholysis typical of psoriasis (a) compared to the straight one (b) typical of traumatic onycholysis.

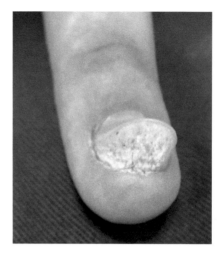

FIGURE 11.4   Subungual hyperkeratosis.

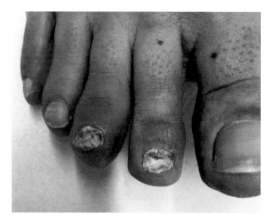

FIGURE 11.5   Dactylitis.

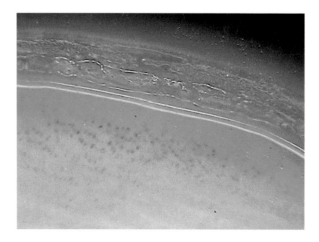

FIGURE 11.6   Hyponychial capillaries.

SUGGESTED READINGS

Chauhan A, Singal A, Grover C, Sharma S. Dermoscopic features of nail psoriasis: an observational, analytical study. *Skin Appendage Disord* 2020;6:207–215.

Haneke E. Nail psoriasis: clinical features, pathogenesis, differential diagnoses, and management. *Psoriasis (Auckl)* 2017;7:51–63.

Iorizzo M, Dahdah M, Vincenzi C, Tosti A. Videodermoscopy of the hyponychium in nail bed psoriasis. *J Am Acad Dermatol* 2008;58:714–715.

CHAPTER 12

Nail Lichen Planus

A S NAIL PSORIASIS, NAIL LICHEN PLANUS IS A BENIGN INFLAMMATORY DISORDER. WHEN the nails are affected, however, it may lead to permanent destruction with severe functional and psychosocial consequences. When the inflammation is limited to the nail matrix, there is altered nail plate formation. Involvement of the proximal nail matrix gives rise to surface alterations, including thinning, fragility, longitudinal ridging, and fissuring. This longitudinal pattern is quite characteristic. In some cases, the matrix is only partially affected. Red spots in the lunula (mottled erythema) also correspond to focal distal matrix inflammation. In more severe cases, matrix involvement may result in marked thinning and shortening of the nail plate with anonychia. Dorsal pterygium is also a sign of severe focal nail matrix involvement with permanent destruction. Nail bed is less commonly affected and usually coexists with nail matrix lichen planus. It is characterized by onycholysis with or without subungual hyperkeratosis. If the onycholysis is severe, the nail plate may be shed resulting in nail bed atrophy (disappearing nail bed syndrome) and permanent anonychia (**Figures 12.1–12.7**).

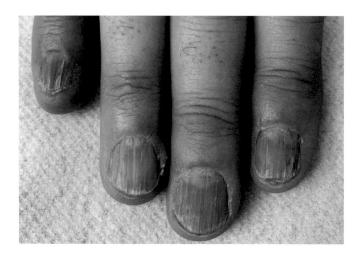

FIGURE 12.1 Typical NLP affecting mostly the matrix with longitudinal ridging and red lunula.

 DOI: 10.1201/b22852-14

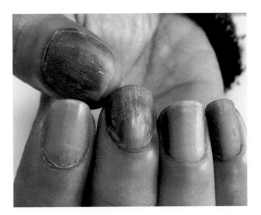

FIGURE 12.2   Typical Nail Lichen Planus (NLP) affecting mostly the bed with onycholysis and subungual hyperkeratosis.

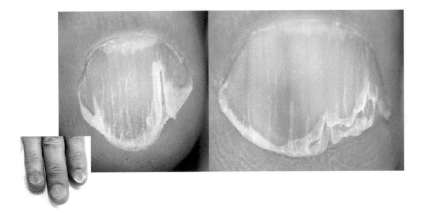

FIGURE 12.3   Typical NLP affecting the matrix with longitudinal splitting and erythronychia.

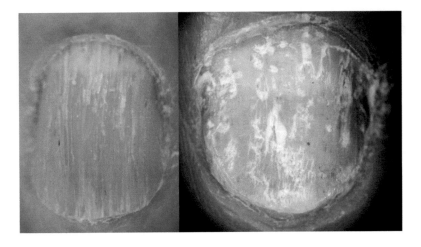

FIGURE 12.4   Typical NLP affecting the matrix with ridging, splinter hemorrhahes and scaling.

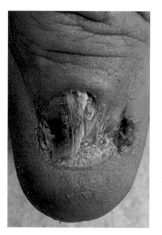 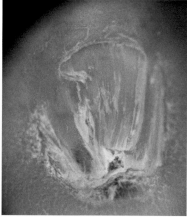

FIGURE 12.5   Typical NLP affecting the matrix with dorsal pterygium.

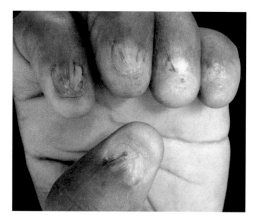

FIGURE 12.6   Typical NLP—severe form/end stage affecting the matrix with anonychia and convergence of the remnant plates to the center of the nail plate.

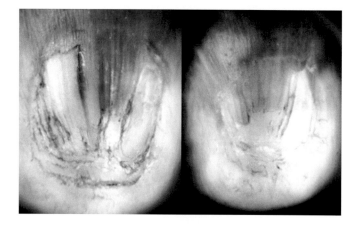

FIGURE 12.7   Typical NLP—severe form/end stage affecting the matrix with anonychia and convergence of the remnant plates to the center of the nail plate (dermoscopy view).

SUGGESTED READINGS

Ceccarelli MA, Gavilanes-Coloma MC, D'almeida L, et al. Description of the most severe signs in nail lichen planus: a strategy to contribute to the diagnosis of the severe stage. *Int J Dermatol* 2022;61:1124–1130.

Grover C, Kharghoria G, Baran R. Nail lichen planus: A review of clinical presentation, diagnosis, and therapy. *Ann Dermatol Venereol* 2022;149:150–164.

Nakamura R, Broce AA, Palencia DP, et al. Dermatoscopy of nail lichen planus. *Int J Dermatol* 2013;52:684–687.

CHAPTER 13

Lichen Striatus

L ICHEN STRIATUS IS A BENIGN, USUALLY UNILATERAL, LINEAR DERMATOSIS TYPICALLY affecting children. It is a cutaneous mosaicism caused by a postzygotic somatic mutation—there is tolerance until a triggering event induces a self-limiting autoimmune T lymphocyte inflammatory reaction. When the nails are affected, typical classic lichenoid nail changes are easily detectable, more often limited to only one portion of the nail or to a single nail plate. It is common to see longitudinal fissuring, onychorrhexis, onycholysis, and subungual hyperkeratosis. Flesh-colored or slightly red flat-topped papules following Blaschko's lines may be associated. The main differential diagnoses are nail lichen planus, nail lichen nitidus, linear nail psoriasis, linear keratosis follicularis, and Inflammatory linear verrucous epidermal nevus (ILVEN). Dermoscopy is an important tool for the diagnosis, but not pathognomonic (**Figures 13.1** and **13.2**).

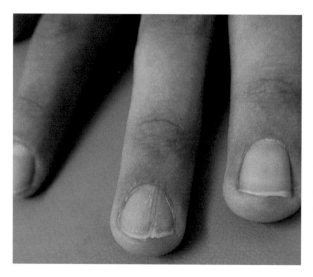 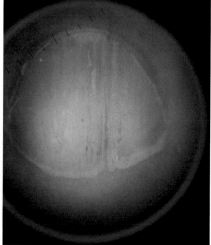

FIGURE 13.1   Nail lichen striatus showing longitudinal erythro-xanthonychia and reddish coloration of the lunular area.

    DOI: 10.1201/b22852-15

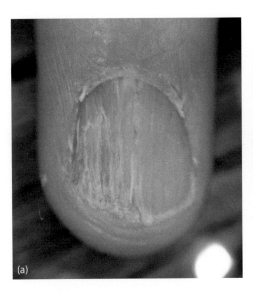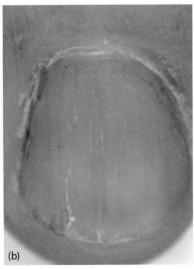

FIGURE 13.2 (a) Nail lichen striatus showing longitudinal splitting and reddish coloration of the lunular area. (b) Same patient healed without treatment after few years.

SUGGESTED READINGS

Iorizzo M, Rubin AI, Starace M. Nail lichen striatus: is dermoscopy useful for the diagnosis? *Pediatr Dermatol* 2019;36:859–863.

Tosti A, Peluso AM, Misciali C, Cameli N. Nail lichen striatus: clinical features and long-term follow-up of five patients. *J Am Acad Dermatol* 1997;36:908–913.

CHAPTER 14

Trachyonychia

THE NAIL PLATE SURFACE IS ROUGH, SANDPAPERED, AND OPAQUE DUE TO INFLAMMATION OF the proximal nail matrix. When the inflammation is mild and intermittent, the result is the shiny variant. Trachyonychia is not specific to nail lichen planus but may also occur in alopecia areata, psoriasis, eczema, and as an idiopathic condition. Pathology is needed for differential diagnosis but, since it is a benign condition, a biopsy is usually not recommended due to its invasiveness and irrelevance to the course of the disease (**Figure 14.1**).

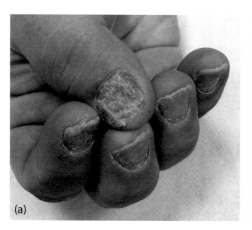 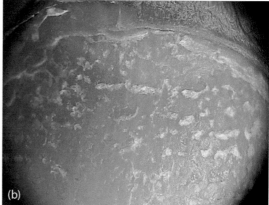

FIGURE 14.1 (a) Clinical and (b) dermoscopy view of trachyonychia where nail plates seem sandpapered.

SUGGESTED READING

Jacobsen AA, Tosti A. Trachyonychia and twenty-nail dystrophy: a comprehensive review and discussion of diagnostic accuracy. *Skin Appendage Disord* 2016;2:7–13.

Starace M, Alessandrini A, Bruni F, Piraccini BM. Trachyonychia: a retrospective study of 122 patients in a period of 30 years. *J Eur Acad Dermatol Venereol*. 2020 Apr;34(4):880–884.

DOI: 10.1201/b22852-16

CHAPTER 15

Warts

Pᴇʀɪᴜɴɢᴜᴀʟ ᴀɴᴅ ꜱᴜʙᴜɴɢᴜᴀʟ ᴡᴀʀᴛꜱ ᴀʀᴇ ᴄᴀᴜꜱᴇᴅ ʙʏ ᴛʜᴇ ʜᴜᴍᴀɴ ᴘᴀᴘɪʟʟᴏᴍᴀᴠɪʀᴜꜱ ᴀɴᴅ are more common in the fingernails than in toenails. They are the most frequent benign tumor of the nail apparatus. Injured or macerated skin is a predisposing condition for their development. Usually, they are cosmetic disturbing but otherwise asymptomatic, though fissuring or subungual localization may cause pain. Consider Bowen disease or squamous cell carcinoma in assumed solitary subungual warts above the age of 40 (**Figures 15.1–15.3**).

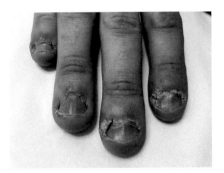

FIGURE 15.1   Multiple periungual warts—not to be confused with ragged cuticles.

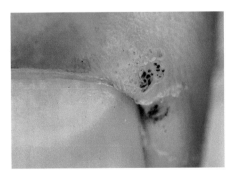

FIGURE 15.2   Differential diagnosis between periungual warts and ragged cuticles/cuticle hyperkeratosis.

DOI: 10.1201/b22852-17

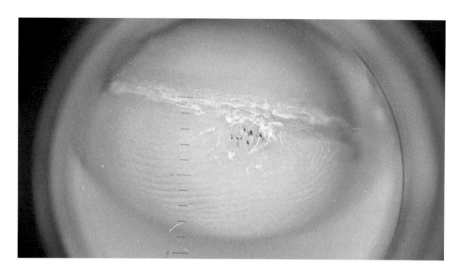

FIGURE 15.3   Dermoscopy allows better visualization of subungual tiny warts.

SUGGESTED READING

Pellacani G, Alessandrini A, Mandel VD, Martella A, Brandi N, Chester J, Piraccini BM, Starace M. Onychoscopy with red light for vascular pattern identification: a study of 33 patients. *J Eur Acad Dermatol Venereol.* 2019 Jul 9.

Subhadarshani S, Sarangi J, Verma KK. Dermoscopy of subungual wart. *Dermatol Pract Concept* 2019;9:22–23.

CHAPTER 16

Bowen Disease/Squamous Cell Carcinoma

SQUAMOUS CELL CARCINOMA (SCC) IS THE MOST FREQUENT MALIGNANT TUMOR OF THE nail apparatus, where presentation as *in situ* SCC (Bowen disease) is more common than invasive SCC.

It is mostly human papillomavirus-related and with a male predominance. Clinically, it may appear as a warty plaque, or even a fibrokeratoma-like lesion, but onycholysis and oozing are the most common presenting signs. Nail plate dystrophy, erythronychia, and pigmentation of the periungual area or the tumor itself may also be observed. *Invasive lesions present with nodules, ulceration, and bleeding.* Diagnosis is often delayed because of the slow evolution of the lesion and multiple clinical features. Intraoperative dermoscopy gives useful information to better approach the diagnosis and to target biopsies—polymorphous vascular structures and whitish scaly areas are usually diagnostic (**Figures 16.1–16.4**).

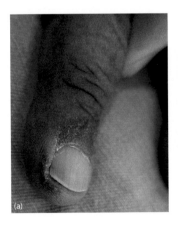
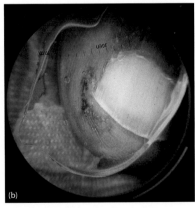

FIGURE 16.1 (a) Pigmented Bowen disease affecting the lateral/distal part of the nail folds. (b) Dermoscopy allows the visualization of whitish scales surrounded by erythematous and brownish pigmentation.

DOI: 10.1201/b22852-18

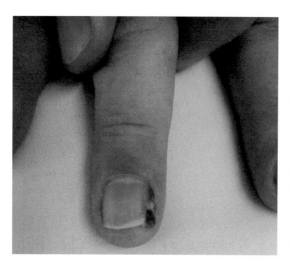 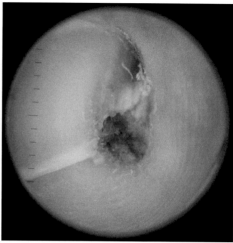

FIGURE 16.2 Pigmented subungual squamous cell carcinoma. Note the pigmented subungual hyperkeratotic mass affecting disto-lateral nail bed.

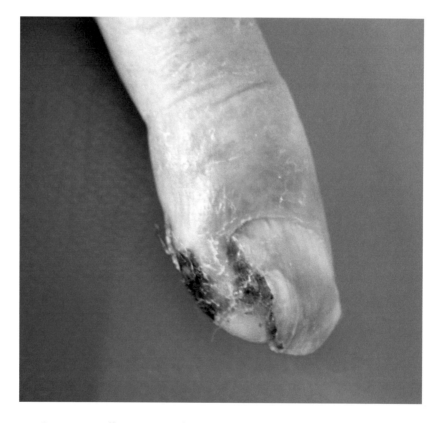

FIGURE 16.3 Squamous cell carcinoma showing a warty lesion and oozing.

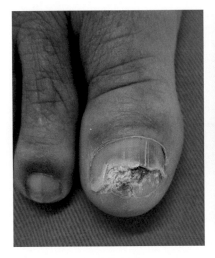 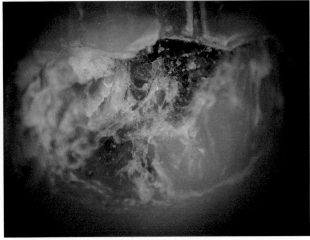

FIGURE 16.4   Invasive squamous cell carcinoma. Although a subungual hyperkeratosis can be seen, some reddish areas are noted only at dermoscopy.

SUGGESTED READINGS

Carlioz V, Perier-Muzet M, Debarbieux S, et al. Intraoperative dermoscopy features of subungual squamous cell carcinoma: a study of 53 cases. *Clin Exp Dermatol* 2021;46:82–88.

Lecerf P, Richert B, Theunis A, André J. A retrospective study of squamous cell carcinoma of the nail unit diagnosed in a Belgian general hospital over a 15-year period. *J Am Acad Dermatol* 2013;69:253–261.

Starace M, Alessandrini A, Dika E, Piraccini BM. Squamous cell carcinoma of the nail unit. *Dermatol Pract Concept.* 2018 Jul 31;8(3):238–244.

CHAPTER 17

Glomus Tumors

GLOMUS TUMOR IS A BENIGN TUMOR ORIGINATING FROM GLOMUS BODIES AND IS MORE frequent in the hand, mainly in the subungual region. It is normally a solitary and painful lesion, seeing through the nail plate as a reddish-blue spot. Usually, the pain is paroxysmal and disproportionate compared to the mild clinical picture. The pain disappears when a tourniquet is applied. Transillumination test, Dermoscopy, Ultrasonography with Doppler, Computed Tomography, and Magnetic Resonance Imaging are useful to define the diagnosis. In some cases, glomus tumor appears as longitudinal erythronychia that does not reach the distal margin, especially in the presence of small masses. Nail plate alterations, such as onycholysis, thinning, and splitting of the nail can also be seen in cases of large masses. Dermoscopy shows paradoxically a whitish nail bed area because of vascular compression by the tumor (**Figure 17.1**).

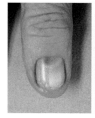 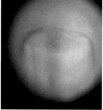 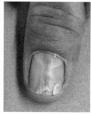 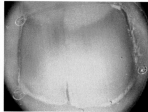 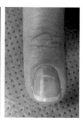

FIGURE 17.1 A glomus tumor in the nail bed can be seen clinically only with difficulty.

SUGGESTED READING

Grover C, Jayasree P, Kaliyadan F. Clinical and onychoscopic characteristics of subungual glomus tumor: a cross-sectional study. *Int J Dermatol* 2021;60:693–702.

Pellacani G, Alessandrini A, Mandel VD, Martella A, Brandi N, Chester J, Piraccini BM, Starace M. Onychoscopy with red light for vascular pattern identification: a study of 33 patients. *J Eur Acad Dermatol Venereol.* 2019

Starace M, Rubin AI, Di Chiacchio NG, Pampaloni F, Alessandrini A, Piraccini BM, Iorizzo M. Diagnosis and surgical treatment of benign nail unit tumors. *J Dtsch Dermatol Ges.* 2023 Feb;21(2):116–129.

 DOI: 10.1201/b22852-19

CHAPTER 18

Acquired Digital Arteriovenous Malformation

IT IS A VASCULAR ALTERATION DUE TO TRAUMA OR FOLLOWING SURGICAL PROCEDURES. Clinically, it appears as a subungual or periungual purple nodule or even as erythronychia. Some benign nail tumors (onychopapilloma, hemangioma, and glomus tumor), as well as malignant ones (Bowen and squamous cell carcinoma), are considered differential diagnoses. Dermoscopy helps to localize and delimitate the lesion. Histopathology confirms the diagnosis (**Figure 18.1**).

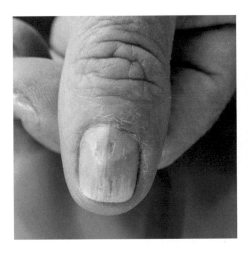 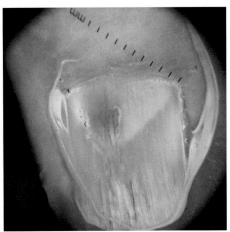

FIGURE 18.1 Acquired digital arteriovenous malformation: clinical aspect with nail ridging, transverse over-curvature of the nail plate, macrolunula with reddish coloration and splinter hemorrhages.

SUGGESTED READING

Kadono T, Kishi A, Onishi Y, Ohara K. Acquired digital arteriovenous malformation: a report of six cases. *Br J Dermatol* 2000;142:362–365.

DOI: 10.1201/b22852-20

CHAPTER 19

Myxoid Pseudocyst

MYXOID OR MUCOID PSEUDOCYSTS ARE A RESULT OF A LEAKAGE OF SYNOVIAL FLUID through a breach in the joint capsule of the interphalangeal joint, as a result of excessive hyaluronic acid production due to osteoarthritis or trauma. They manifest as gradually enlarging cystic-like masses, usually well circumscribed, and localized between the proximal nail fold and the distal interphalangeal joint. Sometimes they discharge gelatinous material.

Clinical features depend upon their location:

- *Type A*: The most common presentation—a nodule between the distal interphalangeal joint and the proximal nail fold.

- *Type B*: A nodule in the proximal nail fold pressing on the underlying matrix resulting in a longitudinal groove in the nail plate.

- *Type C*: A nodule exerting pressure from under the matrix, giving rise to a reddish or bluish lunula.

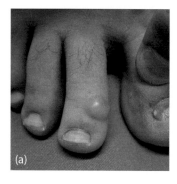 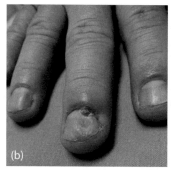 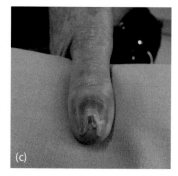

FIGURE 19.1   Myxoid pseudocysts: Clinical aspect of the three different types (a) type A, (b) type B and (c) type C.

    DOI: 10.1201/b22852-21

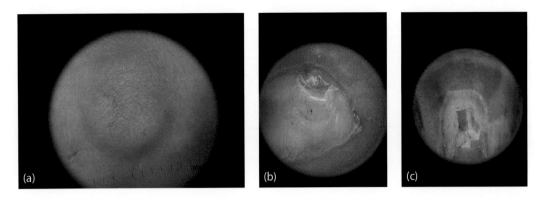

FIGURE 19.2   Myxoid pseudocyst: Dermoscopy of the three different types (a) type A, (b) type B and (c) type C.

Dermoscopy reveals telangiectasias with different patterns (arboriform, polymorphic, punctate, or linear vessels), red-purple lacunas, ulceration, and a bright-whitish reticulum that could be related to an increase in collagen bundles (**Figures 19.1** and **19.2**).

SUGGESTED READING

Güldiken G, Göktay F, Atış G, Güneş P. Evaluation of the demographic and clinical features of patients with digital myxoid pseudocysts and their response to treatment. *Dermatol Surg* 2022;48:625–630.

Starace M, Rapparini L, Quadrelli F, Cedirian S, Pampaloni F, Piraccini BM. *J Eur Acad Dermatol Venereol.* 2024 Mar 9. doi: 10.1111/jdv.19945. Online ahead of print.

CHAPTER 20

Subungual Exostosis

SUBUNGUAL EXOSTOSIS IS A BONY BENIGN TUMOR WITH FIBROUS CARTILAGINOUS CAP arising from the distal phalanx and affecting toenails more often than fingernails. The most common symptom is a painful mass emerging from the nail bed with cosmetic deformity of the nail plate (onycholysis, bulging). Dermoscopy reveals vascular ectasia (neoangiogenesis) as the most common finding, followed by hyperkeratosis of the nail bed and ulceration. A collarette may be present. The hard character of the mass helps to distinguish it from an ungual fibrokeratoma and superficial acral fibromyxoma. X-ray is diagnostic showing an exophytic lesion on the distal phalangeal bone (**Figures 20.1–20.3**).

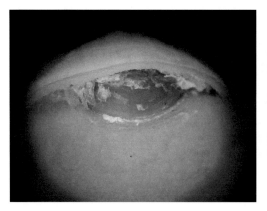 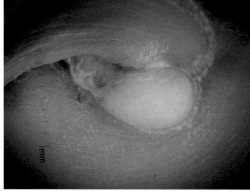

FIGURE 20.1 Subungual exostosis: Subungual hard nodule characterized by vascular ectasia and a collarette delimiting the lesion.

DOI: 10.1201/b22852-22

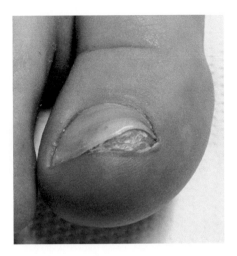

FIGURE 20.2   Subungual exostosis in a child.

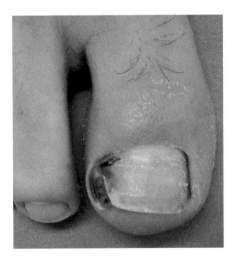

FIGURE 20.3   Exostosis resembling an ingrown toenail.

SUGGESTED READING

Piccolo V, Argenziano G, Alessandrini AM, Russo T, Starace M, Piraccini BM. Dermoscopy of subungual exostosis: a retrospective study of 10 patients. *Dermatology* 2017;233:80–85.

CHAPTER 21

Onychocytic Matricoma

O NYCHOCYTIC MATRICOMA IS A RARE, BENIGN TUMOR OF THE NAIL MATRIX. IT IS considered an acanthoma of the nail matrix that produces onychocytes and, clinically, appears mostly as a longitudinal melanonychia with a corresponding thickened nail plate. It has overlapping histopathologic features with ungual seborrheic keratosis. Because of the clinical presentation, it could mimic a foreign body, but malignancies such as squamous cell carcinoma and melanoma should be ruled out. Due to the possibility of malignant evolution (onychocytic carcinoma), removal should be considered (**Figures 21.1** and **21.2**).

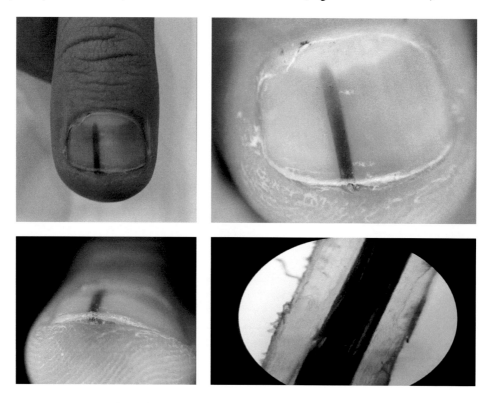

FIGURE 21.1   Pigmented onychocytic matricoma.

DOI: 10.1201/b22852-23

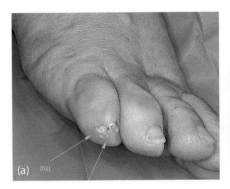 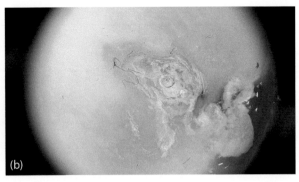

FIGURE 21.2   Onychocytic matricoma (a) clinical view (b) dermoscopy aspect.

SUGGESTED READINGS

Baran R, Moulonguet I, Goettmann-Bonvallot S, et al. Longitudinal subungual acanthoma: one denomination for various clinical presentations. *J Eur Acad Dermatol Venereol* 2018;32:1608–1613.

Wanat KA, Reid E, Rubin AI. Onychocytic matricoma: a new, important nail-unit tumor mistaken for a foreign body. *JAMA Dermatol* 2014; 150:335–337.

CHAPTER 22

Onychomatricoma

ONYCHOMATRICOMA IS A BENIGN NAIL TUMOR THAT ORIGINATES FROM THE NAIL MATRIX. It mainly affects the fingernails and presents with a thickened nail plate (localized or full thickness), over-curvature (transverse and longitudinal), and a whitish/yellow coloration with splinter hemorrhages (xantholeukonychia). Pigmented tumors have been also described. The frontal view of the nail plate shows multiple holes in its thickened free margin (honeycomb holes) corresponding to the digitated fibroepithelial projections of the tumor that grow longitudinally within the nail plate. Onychomycosis is frequently associated, and this often delays the diagnosis. Dermatoscopy shows longitudinal parallel whitish lines, parallel lesion edges, splinter hemorrhages, tortuous hairpin vessels, dark dots, and thickening of the free edge. Observation of the distal margin of the nail plate shows the characteristic holes that make the diagnosis (**Figure 22.1**).

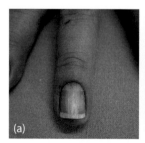 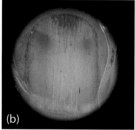 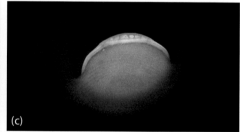

FIGURE 22.1 Onychomatricoma (a) clinical appearance of onychomatricoma: Splinter hemorrhages, thickened nail plate, focal/longitudinal xantonychia, and hypercurvature (transverse and longitudinal). (b) Onychoscopy of the nail plate surface: Yellowish discoloration with longitudinal striae due to the tumor's digitations, which create tunnels and detach the nail plate from the nail bed. Splinter hemorrhages appear as black thin, and short striae due to pinpoint bleeding of nail capillaries and subsequent incorporation of the blood in the ventral nail plate secondary to trauma, especially in thickened nails. (c) The typical dermoscopic aspect in the frontal view is the honeycomb pattern corresponding to the tumor's tunnels excavated within the nail plate. This pattern is represented by white longitudinal grooves analogous to the holes oriented around antero-oblique connective tissue axes.

DOI: 10.1201/b22852-24

SUGGESTED READINGS

Di Chiacchio N, Tavares GT, Tosti A, et al. Onychomatricoma: epidemiological and clinical findings in a large series of 30 cases. *Br J Dermatol* 2015;173:1305–1307.

Lesort C, Debarbieux S, Duru G, et al. Dermoscopic features of onychomatricoma: a study of 34 cases. *Dermatology* 2015;231:177–183.

Starace M, Rubin AI, Di Chiacchio NG, Pampaloni F, Alessandrini A, Piraccini BM, Iorizzo M. Diagnosis and surgical treatment of benign nail unit tumors. *J Dtsch Dermatol Ges.* 2023 Feb;21(2):116–129.

CHAPTER 23

Onychopapilloma

ONYCHOPAPILLOMA IS MOST COMMONLY SEEN IN FINGERNAILS; IT PRESENTS AS A longitudinal band (mostly red but also white or brown), often associated with splinter hemorrhages and a distal splitting of the nail plate. A focal subungual hyperkeratosis or filiform mass is better visualized with dermoscopy of the nail plate free margin. It is painless in 60% of cases but consider removing when painful due to a possible malignant evolution (**Figure 23.1**).

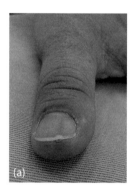 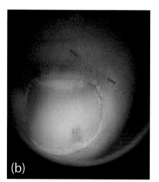 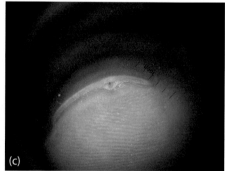

FIGURE 23.1 Onychopapilloma (a) clinical presentation: Longitudinal erythronychia associated with nail plate distal splitting (triangular). (b) Onychoscopy of the nail plate surface: Longitudinal erythronychia associated with a distal triangular splitting of the nail plate. (c) A focal subungual hyperkeratosis is better visualized with onychoscopy of the nail plate's free margin.

SUGGESTED READINGS

Haneke E, Iorizzo M, Gabutti M, Beltraminelli H. Malignant onychopapilloma. *J Cutan Pathol.* 2021 Jan;48(1):174–179.

Starace M, Alessandrini A, Ferrari T, et al. Clinical and onychoscopic features of histopathologically proven onychopapillomas and literature update. *J Cutan Pathol* 2022;49:147–152.

DOI: 10.1201/b22852-25

CHAPTER 24

Subungual Keratoacanthoma

SUBUNGUAL KERATOACANTHOMA IS A BENIGN, RARE, AND RAPIDLY (WITHIN WEEKS) growing painful nodule with a central crater filled with keratin. Underlying bone erosion is common. It is usually located below the free edge of the nail plate or in the most distal portion of the nail bed. The nail plate is usually deformed and irregularly enlarged with superficial fissuring and mild subungual hyperkeratosis, clearly detectable with dermatoscopy (**Figure 24.1**).

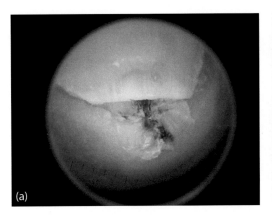
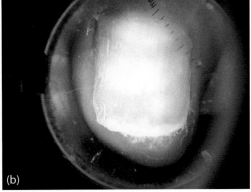

FIGURE 24.1   Subungual keratoacanthoma. (a) Onycholysis and hyperkeratosis of the distal nail bed, associated with hemorrhagic spots. (b) Onycholysis and thiny hyperkeratosis of the distal nail bed, associated with enlargement of the distal nail fold.

SUGGESTED READING

André J, Richert B. Le kératoacanthome sous-unguéal [Subungual keratoacanthoma]. *Ann Dermatol Venereol* 2012;139:68–72.

DOI: 10.1201/b22852-26

CHAPTER 25

Superficial Acral Fibromyxoma

SUPERFICIAL ACRAL FIBROMYXOMA IS A SOFT TISSUE BENIGN TUMOR USUALLY PRESENTING as a flesh-colored slow-growing nodule covered with thin fissured skin. It is usually located in the nail bed or nail folds but exceptionally may be located beneath the matrix. The clinical differential diagnosis includes a cyst, subungual exostosis, and lipoma.

Pain and bone involvement are not frequently observed. Dermoscopy is characterized by polymorphous (curved, arborizing, dotted) vessels, white scar-like patches, shiny white streaks with yellowish hyperkeratotic areas in the center, and finger-like projections with peripheral vascular structures (**Figure 25.1**).

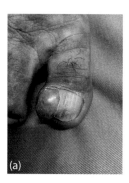 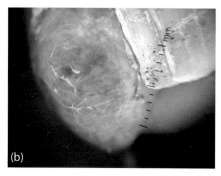

FIGURE 25.1   Superficial acral fibromyxoma. (a) Tumor emerging from the subungual area, with a flesh-colored surface covered with very thin fissured skin. (b) Onychoscopy of the tumor presents as polymorphous vessels with white, scar-like patches, shiny white streaks with yellowish hyperkeratotic areas in the center, and finger-like projections with peripheral vascular structures.

SUGGESTED READING

Starace M, Vezzoni R, Alessandrini A, et al. Superficial acral fibromyxoma: clinical, dermoscopic and histological features of a rare nail tumor. *J Eur Acad Dermatol Venereol* 2023;37:1052–1054.

DOI: 10.1201/b22852-27

CHAPTER 26

Ungual Fibrokeratoma

FIBROKERATOMA IS A SOLITARY AND ASYMPTOMATIC BENIGN FIBROEPITHELIAL TUMOR that forms in the periungual area or within or under the nail plate. It shows distally a hyperkeratotic tip that helps in the differential diagnosis of fibroma. Depending on the location, nail plate dystrophies may be associated. Dermoscopy reveals a central homogeneous pale-yellow area surrounded by a hyperkeratotic white scaly collarette. The presence of clumps of homogenous red lacunae divided by white meshwork-like keratotic septa with telangiectasia on the adjacent skin has also been reported (**Figure 26.1**).

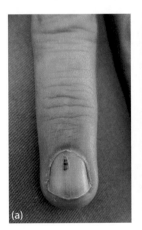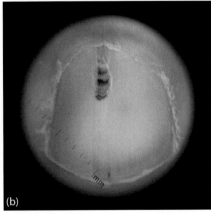

FIGURE 26.1 Ungual fibrokeratoma. (a) Longitudinal canalicular depression of the nail plate associated with a yellowish filiform tumor emerging from the cuticle. (b) Onychoscopy reveals focal hyperkeratosis on the distal part of the tumor, tortuous vessels on its proximal part, and transverse hemorrhages affecting the lesion.

SUGGESTED READING

Shih S, Khachemoune A. Acquired digital fibrokeratoma: review of its clinical and dermoscopic features and differential diagnosis. *Int J Dermatol* 2019;58:151–158.

Starace M, Rapparini L, Quadrelli F, Cedirian S, Pampaloni F, Piraccini BM. *J Eur Acad Dermatol Venereol*. 2024 Mar 9. doi: 10.1111/jdv.19945. Online ahead of print.

DOI: 10.1201/b22852-28

CHAPTER 27

Ungual Fibroma

THIS CAN APPEAR AS A PERIUNGUAL OR SUBUNGUAL BENIGN TUMOR CLASSICALLY associated with tuberous sclerosis (Koenen's tumor). No histological difference has been found between isolated acquired ungual fibrokeratomas and Koenen's tumors, although the latter has no prominent hyperkeratotic tip (**Figure 27.1**).

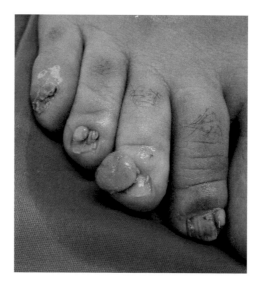

FIGURE 27.1 Ungual fibroma: Multiple fibroma affecting the periungual area on a patient with sclerosis tuberosa.

SUGGESTED READING

Oba MÇ, Uzunçakmak TK, Sar M, et al. Dermoscopic findings in a case of multiple subungual fibromas. *Acta Dermatovenerol Alp Pannonica Adriat* 2021;30:35–37.

DOI: 10.1201/b22852-29

CHAPTER 28

Longitudinal Melanonychia

L ONGITUDINAL MELANONYCHIA (LM) DESCRIBES THE PRESENCE OF MELANIN WITHIN the nail plate in longitudinal bands due to melanocyte activation or a benign (lentigo, nevus) or malignant melanocyte hyperplasia (melanoma).

When dealing with melanonychia, it is always advisable to first consider various causes of activation, including ethnicity, drug intake, or an inflammatory/infective disorder (e.g., lichen planus, paronychia, onychomycosis, onychotillomania). The importance of diagnosing melanonychia—still a challenge for general physicians and dermatologists—is recognizing the early stages of nail melanoma.

Clinical features considered worrisome in adults are:

- *Hutchinson sign*: an extension of the pigmentation to the nail folds. It is a presumptive but not pathognomonic sign of nail melanoma;

- *Nail plate dystrophy*: fissuring, splitting, localized thinning;

- *Distal narrowing of the pigmented band*: it indicates that the lesion is increasing proximally;

- The central part of the lesion is dark and its lateral part is clearer and blurred (lines not homogeneous in color, spacing, and thickness with disrupted parallelism);

- Vascular abnormalities and ulcerations of the nail tissues (bed/periungual area).

When observed in children, these worrisome signs are rarely associated with malignancy.

Dermoscopy is an essential tool for diagnosis and can be performed on the nail plate and even intraoperative, allowing a better view of the origin of the pigmented lesion.

NAIL PLATE DERMOSCOPY

Grayish LM typically means melanocytic activation and brownish to black color means melanocytic hyperplasia (nevi, lentigo, or melanoma). Longitudinal lines must be observed according to their regularity, considering the spacing between them,

DOI: 10.1201/b22852-30

parallelism, thickness, and color variation. A regular pattern indicates a benign lesion, while an irregular pattern suggests malignancy. When the nail plate is thick, or the pigmentation is intense, the longitudinal lines cannot be observed and do not allow definitive conclusions.

INTRAOPERATIVE DERMOSCOPY

It is indicated in suspicious cases when a biopsy is mandatory. The view of the origin of the pigment permits better conclusion compared to observation of the plate only. Reclining the proximal nail fold and removing the proximal third of the nail plate is necessary for a direct view of the pigmented lesion.

Color and lines are evaluated, showing four different patterns:

- Regular and thin lines grayish in color are often observed in cases of melanocytic activation (*hypermelanosis*).

- Regular lines brownish in color are suggestive of *lentigo*.

- Regular lines brownish in color plus dots and blotches indicate *nevi*.

- Irregular lines in color and thickness suggest *melanoma*.

Although dermoscopy is a helpful tool in the diagnosis of melanonychia and nail melanoma, histopathological examination of the pigmented lesion is still considered the gold standard (**Figure 28.1–28.12**).

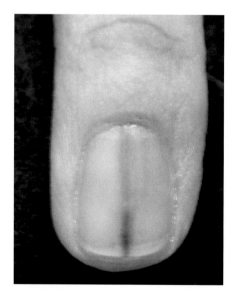

FIGURE 28.1 Worrisome feature: The medial part of the lesion dark, and lateral clearer and blurred.

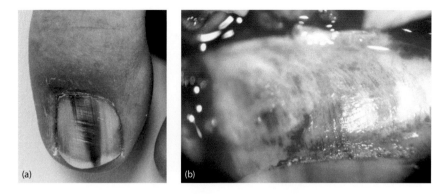

FIGURE 28.2 *In situ* melanoma: Triangular shape: (a) The base of the triangle in the proximal nail fold, indicating the radial growth of the pigmented matrix lesion. (b) Intraoperative dermoscopy shows irregular brown bands in the distal matrix.

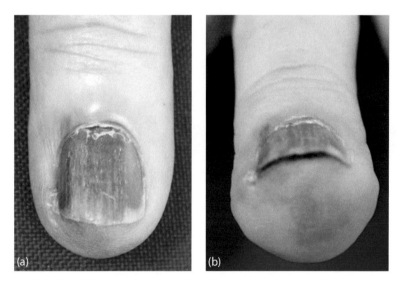

FIGURE 28.3 Hutchinson's sign: (a) Proximal and (b) distal fold pigmentation.

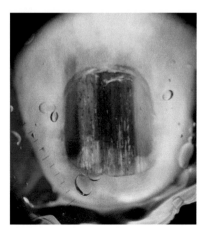

FIGURE 28.4 Hutchinson's sign: Dermoscopy aspects.

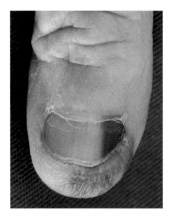

FIGURE 28.5   Hutchinson's sign: Pigmentation of distal and lateral folds.

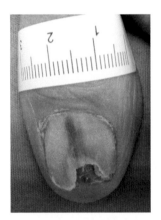 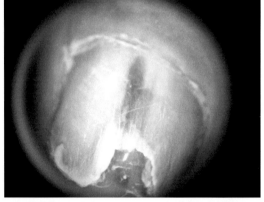

FIGURE 28.6   Worrisome feature: Nail plate dystrophy.

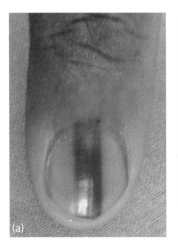 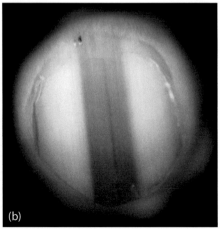

FIGURE 28.7   Nevus in adult. (a) Clinical view showing a homogeneous brown band and pseudo Hutchinson's sign. (b) Dermoscopy of the nail plate shows regular brown lines and a hyperpigmented central line.

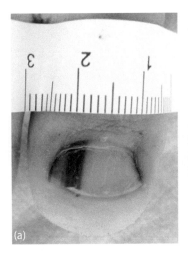
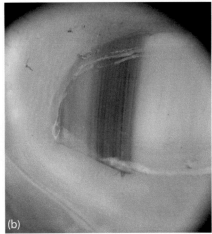

FIGURE 28.8 Nevus in a child. (a) Clinical view showing a large (5 mm) brown band, with different hues of pigmentation (light, dark brown, and black), pseudo and true Hutchinson's sign. (b) Dermoscopy of the nail plate shows regular and irregular brown lines.

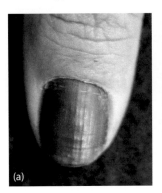
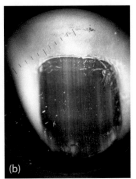
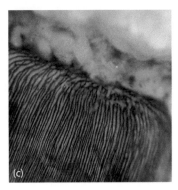

FIGURE 28.9 (a) Melanonychia: Lentigo: Total black nail. (b) Dermoscopy of nail plate: Difficult to see the lines due to excess melanin pigment. (c) Intraoperative dermoscopy exhibiting parallel and regular brown lines.

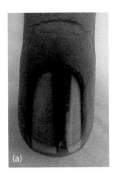
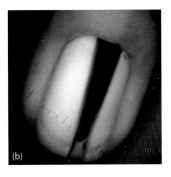
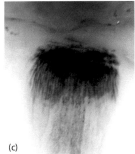

FIGURE 28.10 *In situ* melanoma: (a) Band with triangular shape and distal nail dystrophy. (b) Dermoscopy of nail plate: Irregular lines with different hue of pigmentation. (c) Intraoperative dermoscopy exhibiting irregular lines and blotches.

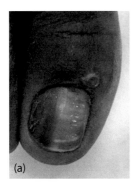 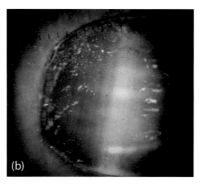 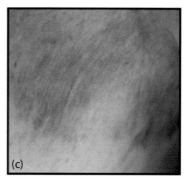

FIGURE 28.11   Hypermelanosis: (a) Clinical aspect: Light brown band. (b) Dermoscopy of nail plate: Light brown color—difficult to see lines. (c) Intraoperative dermoscopy visualization of gray/light brown and regular thin lines.

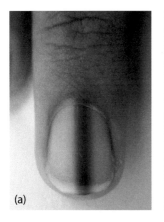 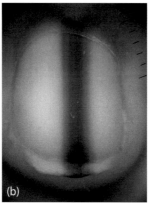 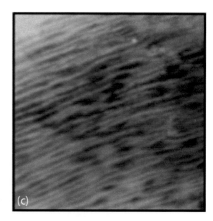

FIGURE 28.12   Nevi: (a) Clinical aspect: A brown longitudinal nail band. (b) Dermoscopy of nail plate: Light brown and regular lines with a central dark brown line. (c) Intraoperative dermoscopy evidencing regular brown lines with blotches and dots.

SUGGESTED READINGS

Clinical and dermoscopic clues to differentiate pigmentes nail bands: an International Dermoscopy Society study. Benati E, Ribero S, Longo C, Piana S, Puig S, Carrera C, Cicero F, Kittler H, Deinlein T, Zalaudek I, Stolz W, Scope A, Pellacani G, Moscarella E, Piraccini BM, Starace M, Argenziano G. *J Eur Acad Dermatol Venereol*. 2016 Oct 1.

Hirata SH, Yamada S, Enokihara MY, et al. Patterns of nail matrix and bed of longitudinal melanonychia by intraoperative dermatoscopy. *J Am Acad Dermatol* 2011;65:297–303.

Longo C, Pampena R, Moscarella E, Chester J, Starace M, Cinotti E, Piraccini, BM, Argenziano G, Peris K, Pellacani G. Dermoscopy of melanoma according to different body sites: Head and neck, trunk, limbs, nail, mucosal and acral. *J Eur Acad Dermatol Venereol*. 2023 May 21.

Nail apparatus melanoma: dermoscopic and histopathologi correlations on a series of 23 patients from a single centre.

Ohn J, et al. Dermoscopic features of nail matrix nevus (NMN) in adults and children: a comparative analysis. *J Am Acad Dermatol* 2016;75:535–540.

Starace M, Dika E, Fanti PA, Patrizi A, Misciali C, Alessandrini A, Bruni F, Piraccini BM. *J Eur Acad Dermatol Venereol*. 2017 Aug 29.

CHAPTER 29

Leishmaniasis

Cutaneous leishmaniasis is endemic in many countries, but nail unit involvement has rarely been reported. It is caused by an intracellular protozoan of the genus Leishmania, which is frequent in fingers, although it was also described in the great toe. The lesion appears as a chronic paronychia, ulceration, or may even be verrucous. Patients who live or have visited endemic areas with other skin lesions suggestive and unresponsive to antibiotic therapy are suspicious. Slit-skin smear, biopsy, and molecular diagnostic tests confirm the diagnosis.

Although no dermoscopy findings of nail leishmaniasis are described in the literature, the cutaneous disease may present erythema, hyperkeratosis with central erosion or ulceration, white scar-like patch, yellow tears, white starburst sign, milia-like cyst, and irregular vascular structures (**Figure 29.1**).

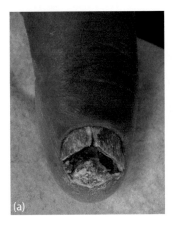 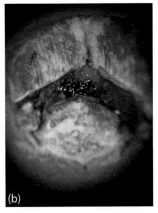

FIGURE 29.1   (a) Onycholysis associated with nail thinning, medial-proximal nail bed erosion, and distal nail bed hyperkeratosis. (b) Nail bed erosion and hyperkeratosis of the distal nail bed.

SUGGESTED READING

Oguz Topal I, Duman H, Baz V, et al. Pediatric dermatology photoquiz: refractory purulent paronychia in a young girl. Paronychial cutaneous leishmaniasis. *Pediatr Dermatol* 2016;33:93–4.

DOI: 10.1201/b22852-31

CHAPTER 30

Leprosy

NAIL CHANGES IN PATIENTS WITH LEPROSY (LEPROMATOUS OR TUBERCULOID) ARE frequent, not specific, but a sign of trophic changes and a clue for the diagnosis. Trauma, neuropathy, vasculopathy, drugs reaction, and infections are the main causes of nail alterations.

Oncholysis, onychogryphosis, hapalonychia, pitting, nail pallor, leukonychia, melanonychia, subungual hematoma, onychauxis, thinning, longitudinal splits, atrophy, and anonychia are all nail changes observed in leprosy patients. Bone involvement is usually severe (**Figure 30.1**).

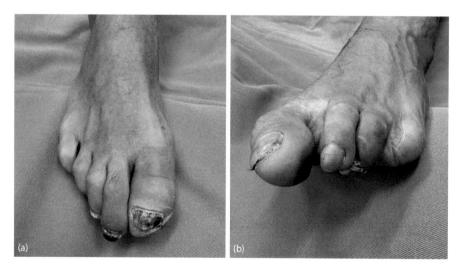

FIGURE 30.1 Nail alteration due to leprosy (melanonychia, onychomycosis, haematoma, and transverse overcurvature of the nail) (a) Right foot. (b) Left foot.

SUGGESTED READING

Rajput CD, Nikam BP, Gore SB, Malani SS. Nail changes in leprosy: an observational study of 125 patients. *Indian Dermatol Online J* 2020;11:195–201.

 DOI: 10.1201/b22852-32

CHAPTER 31

Tungiasis

*T*UNGA PENETRANS IS MORE ASSOCIATED WITH HUMAN INFECTIONS AND IS ENDEMIC IN Latin America, the Caribbean, and Africa. Tungiasis is more common in feet and legs. It can be observed in the interdigital area, calcaneal area, plantar region, proximal and lateral nail folds, and subungual region. It is characterized by a whitish papule surrounded by erythema and a central, dark point. When the flea dies, the lesion involutes, and a blackish crust appears as a residual lesion.

Onychoscopy can improve the visualization of *Tunga penetrans* and the peripheral ring corresponding to the flea's abdomen and the parasite's posterior segment (**Figure 31.1**).

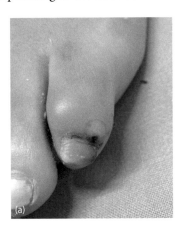
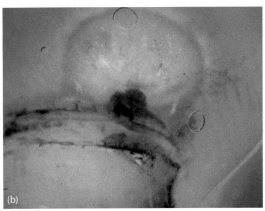

FIGURE 31.1 (a) Clinical aspect shows a yellowish bulla affecting the proximal nail fold with a black dot on the cuticle. (b) Onychoscopy allows the visualization of the peripheral ring corresponding to the flea's abdomen and the parasite's posterior segment in the cuticula/proximal nail fold.

SUGGESTED READINGS

Flajoliet N, Bertolotti A. Potential use of dermoscopy in atypical tungiasis. *J Travel Med* 2021;28:taab072.

Noriega L, Di Chiacchio N, Rosa IP, et al. Subungual hyperpigmented nodular lesion in an adult's toe. *Skin Appendage Disord* 2016;1:114–116.

DOI: 10.1201/b22852-33

Index